RENAL DIET FOR A HEALTHY FAMILY

3 BOOKS in 1: The Ultimate Diet to Control Kidney Disease with a Low Sodium, Low Potassium, Low Phosphorus Meal Plan. With 350+ Delicious Renal-Friendly Recipes

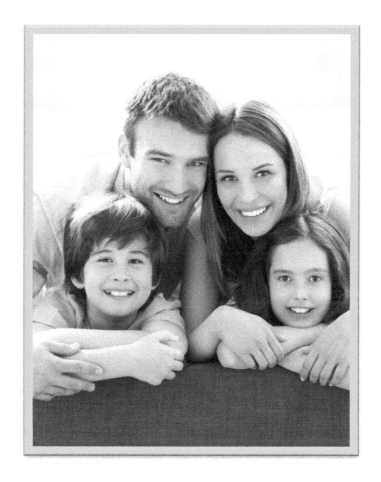

By

MELISSA SIMPSON, M.D.

TABLE OF CONTENT

PART I: INTRODUCTION

A kidney diet is a diet that is prescribed to diabetic patients to control their urine production. You need to know the term of renal diet to follow this diet and be easily manipulated to improve diabetic problems.

Usually, the kidney of any patient is not working as per the requirement, it is working under the condition, and this lack of function is hazardous for the body. In short, it is known as kidney failure. Therefore, people suffering from this problem need to have a proper checkup to learn to see the extent of the problem. If a good checkup is done, it can be easily detected.

So, it is better to know what a renal diet is and how to do it, how to treat the disease, and how to make the kidney work properly.

A renal diet is also known as a "diabetic diet." As the kidney of a diabetic patient is not function correctly, this diet helps to control the urine production of the diabetic patient. So, this diet is beneficial in the case of a diabetic patient. Even if the patient has diabetes, still the doctor will recommend him to do this diet. This is because this diet helps to control the amount of sugar that is excreted in the urine. By controlling the excretion of sugar in the urine, the patient can have fewer complications caused by diabetes.

According to some specialists, renal diet is beneficial only in diabetic patients. A patient who has cancer, kidney disease, heart disease, lung disease should not follow a kidney diet because it will weaken his physical condition.

The unique thing about the kidney diet is the kind of food that is good for healthy kidneys. If a person suffers from some disease in typical cases, he can recover quickly if he has a proper diet. If there is some deficiency in the kidney, some problems with this kidney cannot work correctly for all people; some people may work correctly. But the kidney problem will be severe because of diabetes.

A kidney is a place where a lot of was it purifies and extracts all the waste and impurities from the body. So, it is a vital organ of the human body. So, if this organ is not working correctly, the body will not be able to function correctly.

To decrease the amount of waste in the blood, individuals with impaired kidney function must adhere to a kidney diet. Waste in the blood is produced by liquids and foods that are ingested. Because kidney activity is impaired, the kidneys do not adequately filter or extract the waste. If the excess remains in the blood, it negatively affects the patient's electrolyte levels. Maintaining a renal diet can help improve kidney function and delay the progression of kidney failure.

A diet deficient in phosphorus, protein, and sodium is a renal diet. A renal diet often emphasizes the value of consuming high-quality protein and typically limits fluids. Calcium and potassium will also need to be modified for specific patients. An individual's body is different, so each patient needs to work with a renal dietitian to create a diet customized to the patient's needs.

Substances that are essential for screening to support a renal diet are listed below:

Sodium

What is the role of sodium in the body?

In particular natural foods, sodium is a mineral that is present. Most individuals think of sodium and salt as synonymous. However, salt is a complex of sodium and chloride. Therefore, the food we consume may include salt, which may contain other sources of sodium. Because of the added salt, refined foods also produce higher levels of sodium.

Sodium is one of the three main electrolytes in the body (chloride and potassium are the other two). Electrolytes regulate the fluids that enter and leave the body's tissues and cells. Sodium contributes to:

- Regulating nerve activity and muscle contraction
- Controlling blood volume and blood pressure
- Balancing the amount of fluid stored or eliminated from the body
- Regulating the acid-base balance of the blood

Why should renal patients monitor their sodium intake?

When fluid and sodium build up in the bloodstream and tissues, it can cause:

- Edema: swelling of the hands, face, and legs
- Increased thirst
- Shortness of breath: fluid builds up in the lungs, making it difficult to breathe.
- Heart failure: The heart will work too hard with the extra fluid in the bloodstream, making it weak and enlarged.
- High blood pressure

How can patients control their sodium intake?

- For portion sizes, be very careful.
- Always read the label on the food. Always list the sodium content.
- Choose fresh vegetables and fruits or frozen and canned products with no added salt.
- Use fresh meat instead of packaged meat.
- Compare brands and use those with the lowest sodium content.
- Avoid processed products.
- Prepare at home and do NOT add salt.
- Use spices that do not have "salt" in the title (prefer garlic powder instead of garlic salt).
- Limit total sodium level per meal to 400 mg and per snack to 150 mg.

Potassium

In maintaining a regular heartbeat and proper muscle function, potassium plays an important role. The kidneys help keep the correct amount of potassium in the body and remove excess amounts in the urine.

Why should patients with kidneys monitor their potassium intake?

High potassium in the blood is known as hyperkalemia which can trigger

- An abnormal heartbeat
- Weakness in the muscles
- Death
- Heart attacks
- Slow pulse

How can patients control their potassium intake?

In some foods, phosphorus can be identified. Therefore, to better control amounts of phosphorus, patients with impaired kidney function can consult a renal dietitian.

Tips to help keep phosphorus at healthy levels:

- For portion sizes, pay close attention to.
- Know which foods have less phosphorus.
- Eating fresh fruits and vegetables.
- Eat small amounts of protein-rich foods for snacks and meals.
- Avoid packaged foods that contain added phosphorus. On ingredient labels, look for phosphorus and words with "PHOS" in them.
- Ask your doctor about using phosphate binders with meals.
- Keep a food diary

Protein

Protein is usually absorbing waste products are produced that are purified by the nephrons of the kidneys. Then, the waste is turned into the urine with the help of other kidney proteins. But, on the other hand, damaged kidneys refuse to eliminate protein waste, and it accumulates in the blood.

For patients with chronic kidney disorders, adequate protein intake is derrick. The amount varies depending on the level of the disease. Protein is necessary for tissue maintenance and other bodily roles. Still, according to the renal dietitian or nephrologist, it is essential to consume the amount prescribed for the particular stage of the disease.

Fluids

For patients in the later stages of kidney disease, fluid management is essential because regular fluid intake can contribute to fluid build-up in the body that can become detrimental. People on dialysis also have a reduced flow of urine, so the additional fluid in the body will put undue pressure on the person's lungs and heart.

Based on urine output and dialysis conditions, a patient's fluid allocation is measured individually. Therefore, asking the nephrologist/nutritionist for fluid intake guidelines is essential.

To monitor fluid intake, patients should:

- Do not drink more than prescribed by the physician.
- Count all foods that dissolve at room temperature.
- Know the number of fluids used for cooking.

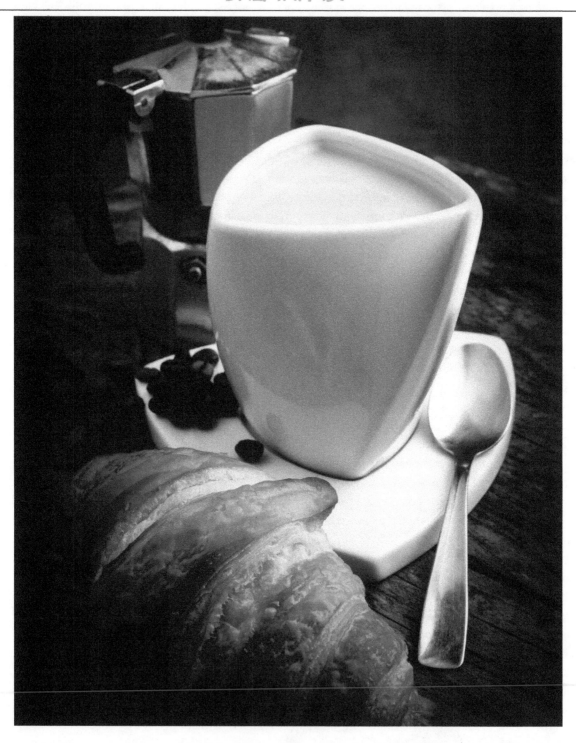

1) Muffins with spinach

Preparation Time: 10 min   **Cooking Time**: none   **Servings: 6**

Ingredients:
- ✓ Six eggs
- ✓ 1/2 cup fat-free milk
- ✓ 1 cup of low-fat crumbled cheese
- ✓ Spinach 4 ounces

Directions:
- ❖ Integrate eggs with milk, cheese, spinach and red spinach in a dish. Mix well with pepper and ham.

Ingredients:
- ✓ 1/2 cup of roasted red bell pepper, chopped
- ✓ Ham Two ounces, sliced
- ✓ Spray firing

- ❖ Oil a muffin pan with cooking spray, divide muffin mix, place in oven and bake for thirty minutes at 350 degrees Fahrenheit
- ❖ Divide the plates and serve them for breakfast. Enjoy!

2) Bowl of blueberry smoothie

Preparation Time: 15-20 min   **Cooking Time**: 15 min   **Servings: 1**

Ingredients:
- ✓ 2 tablespoons of shredded coconut
- ✓ 1 tablespoon of fiber cereal
- ✓ 2 strawberries
- ✓ 5 raspberries

Directions:
- ❖ In a blender, mix the blueberries
- ❖ Add the yogurt, milk and protein powder and mix until smooth.

Ingredients:
- ✓ 1/3 cup unsweetened vanilla almond milk
- ✓ ¼ cup of fat-free Greek yogurt
- ✓ 2 tablespoons of whey protein powder
- ✓ 1 cup blueberries, frozen
- ❖ Place the mixture in a bowl and top it off with some chopped raspberries, strawberries, cereal and coconut.

3) Egg white omelette with vegetables

Preparation Time: 10 min   **Cooking Time**: 10 min   **Servings: 2**

Ingredients:
- ✓ Six white eggs
- ✓ One tablespoon of water
- ✓ Two tablespoons of olive oil
- ✓ 1/2 yellow onion, sliced

Directions:
- ❖ In a medium bowl, beat egg whites, insert 1 tablespoon water and stir. With a fork until well blended.
- ❖ Heat 1 teaspoon oil in a medium-sized skillet over medium-high heat. Add the onions, tomatoes, asparagus and mushrooms and sauté until the vegetables are tender about 3-4 minutes. Remove from the skillet and dismiss.
- ❖ Introduce another teaspoon of oil into the skillet and allow it to heat for a minute or two. Bring the beaten eggs into the pan, swirling the pan as required so that the eggs cover the entire pan.

Ingredients:
- ✓ 1 sliced tomato
- ✓ 2-3 asparagus stalks, cut into small pieces
- ✓ 3-4 cut mushrooms

- ❖ Let the eggs settle along the edges of the pan, it will only take a few moments if the pan is hot enough. Using a spatula, slide the eggs away from the edges of the pan and turn the pan to allow the egg mixture to circulate over the surface of the pan. Repeat until the eggs are almost done but still soft in the center.
- ❖ Introduce the vegetable mixture into the center of the omelet. Fold one side of the omelet over the toppings. Slide onto a plate. Voila, it's safe to serve.

4) Breakfast salad with fruit and yogurt

Preparation Time: 10 min   **Cooking Time**: 15-20 min   **Servings: 6**

Ingredients:

- ✓ 2 cups of water
- ✓ 1/4 teaspoon salt
- ✓ 3/4 cup of quick-cooking brown rice
- ✓ 3/4 cup bulgur
- ✓ One large apple, peeled and diced

Directions:

- ❖ Heat water over high heat in a large pot until it boils.
- ❖ Integrate the salt, rice and bulgur into the mixture. Reduce heat, cover and simmer for ten minutes. Remove from heat and encourage to sit for 2 minutes, covered.

Ingredients:

- ✓ One large pear, peeled and chopped
- ✓ One orange, peeled and cut into pieces
- ✓ 1 cup dried cranberries
- ✓ 1 box (8 ounces) of low-fat or fat-free plain Greek yogurt
- ❖ Place the grains in a large bowl and chill in the refrigerator until chilled.
- ❖ Take cold grains out of the freezer. Add strawberries, pears, bananas Cranberries that are dry. Fold and gently whisk in yogurt until grains and fruit are set. Wrap completely.
- ❖ In bowls, serve.

5) Spiced pumpkin fritters

Preparation Time: 5 min   **Cooking Time**: 10 min   **Servings: 10**

Ingredients:

- ✓ Two cups of total wheat flour
- ✓ Two teaspoons of flour for cooking
- ✓ One teaspoon of cooking soda
- ✓ One teaspoon of cinnamon
- ✓ 1/2 teaspoon of nutmeg
- ✓ 1/2 teaspoon ground ginger

Directions:

- ❖ Mix flour, baking powder, baking powder and baking soda together in a mixing bowl. 2. Nutmeg, cinnamon and ginger.
- ❖ Mix brown sugar, egg yolk and pumpkin in another dish. Stir in the milk.
- ❖ Pour the milk mixture with the dry ingredients into a pan. Stir until just melted. Do not over stir.

Ingredients:

- ✓ 1/4 cup brown sugar
- ✓ 1 egg yolk
- ✓ One cup of canned pumpkin
- ✓ Two tablespoons of coconut oil
- ✓ Skimmed milk Two cups
- ✓ Two egg whites
- ❖ In a skillet, beat egg whites until smooth. Fold the egg whites into the pancake batter.
- ❖ Over moderate heat, heat a nonstick skillet or large frying pan. Sprinkle with nonstick cooking.
- ❖ When the griddle is heated, 1/4 cup of ladle batter is applied to the pan. Cook for a while before the batter begins to bubble, flip, and cook until gently browned.

6) Lemon and zucchini muffins

Preparation Time: 5 min   **Cooking Time**: 10 min   **Servings: 12**

Ingredients:
- ✓ All-purpose flour - 2 cups
- ✓ 1/2 of a cup of sugar
- ✓ 1 tablespoon of flour for cooking
- ✓ 1/4 teaspoon salt
- ✓ 1/4 teaspoon of cinnamon
- ✓ 1/4 cup nutmeg

Directions:
- ❖ Preheat oven to 400°F. By gently spraying, ready the muffin tray or cooking spray or muffin liner.
- ❖ Integrate the flour, sugar, baking powder, salt, cinnamon, etc. into a blender bowl with the nutmeg.

Ingredients:
- ✓ 1 cup shredded zucchini
- ✓ 3/4 cup of fat-free milk
- ✓ Olive oil, 2 teaspoons
- ✓ Lemon juice for 2 tablespoons
- ✓ egg
- ✓ Non-stick mist for cooking
- ❖ Integrate the zucchini, milk, oil, lemon juice and egg into another dish. Mix well.
- ❖ Apply the zucchini solution to the flour combination. Stir before they are all mixed. Do not over mix.
- ❖ On the packaged muffin cups, add the batter. Bake for 20 minutes or until lightly browned.

7) English Muffin Breakfast

Preparation Time: 5 min   **Cooking Time**: 8 min   **Servings: 1**

Ingredients:
- ✓ 1⁄2 whole wheat English muffin
- ✓ One piece of low-fat Swiss cheese (2% milk), cut into pieces to fit the muffin Olive oil in a sprayer with pumps

Directions:
- ❖ Toast the English muffin in a grill or microwave toaster. Turn off the toaster
- ❖ Cover muffin with cheese slices and let stand until cheese begins to melt from heat generated for about 30 seconds. Move to a plate.
- ❖ Meanwhile, brush oil into a small nonstick skillet and cook over medium heat.
- ❖ Apply the egg substitute and bake for about 15 seconds before securing the edges.

Ingredients:
- ✓ 1⁄2 cup of seasoned egg substitute liquid
- ✓ 11⁄2 teaspoons coarsely diced shallots (green part only)
- ❖ Using a heat-resistant spatula, lift the sides of the egg substitute so that the uncooked liquid underneath flows out. Continue to cook, lifting the sides about every 15 seconds before the egg combination is done, for a total of 11⁄2 minutes. Using the spatula,
- ❖ To produce a sturdy "patty," fold the sides of the beaten egg into the core about 2 inches wide.

8) Tartlets with strawberries and cream cheese 1

Preparation Time: 5 min   **Cooking Time**: 10 min   **Servings**: 1

Ingredients:
- ✓ A slice of wholemeal bread
- ✓ Two tablespoons of fat-free spreadable cheese

Directions:
- ❖ In a toaster oven, toast the bread.

Ingredients:
- ✓ Two large strawberries cut into pieces
- ✓ Honey for 1 teaspoon (optional)
- ❖ Layer with the cream cheese and finish with the cream cheese on top of the strawberries.

9) Broccoli and Pepper Jack Omelette

Preparation Time: 5 min   **Cooking Time**: 10 min   **Servings**: 1

Ingredients:
- ✓ In a pump sprayer, olive oil
- ✓ 1/2 cup of seasoned egg substitute liquid

Directions:
- ❖ Drizzle a small nonstick skillet over medium heat with oil and heat. Add the eggs, then
- ❖ Reposition and bake for about 15 seconds before the edges are set. Use a heat-resistant spatula
- ❖ Lift the edges of the egg substitute so that the uncooked liquid flows underneath.

Ingredients:
- ✓ A low-fat pepper jack cheese (2% milk) cut, torn into a few 1/4 cup pieces
- ✓ Broccoli (thawed frozen ones are fine), fried and sliced, reheated in the microwave,
- ❖ Continue to cook, lifting the sides every 15 seconds or so, until the omelet is done, about 1 1/2 minutes total.
- ❖ Remove from heat. Spread the rest of the cheese and broccoli omelet on top. Turn the pan marginally and use the spatula to fold the omelet again and again and into thirds. (From the heat of the omelet, the cheese will melt).
- ❖ Slide out. Place on a tray and then serve.

10) Granola your way

Preparation Time: 5 min   **Cooking Time**: 7 min   **Servings**: 10

Ingredients:
- ✓ 1/4 cup medium brown sugar, rolled
- ✓ Two tablespoons of water
- ✓ One tablespoon of oil for the vegetables
- ✓ One teaspoon of cinnamon powder
- ✓ One tablespoon of maple extract or vanilla flavoring
- ✓ Four cups old-fashioned oats (rolled)

Directions:
- ❖ Mix brown sugar, water, oil, cinnamon and maple in a large dish.
- ❖ Flavor until sugar is dissolved. Insert oats and whisk in once lightly covered. On a large cookie sheet, spread evenly.
- ❖ Bake, stirring regularly and pushing the toasted sides into the center of the Granola, for about 40 minutes, until the oats are evenly crisp.

Ingredients:
- ✓ One cup of medium grapes
- ✓ 1/2 cup chopped dates
- ✓ 1/2 cup milk, fat-free, to serve
- ✓ Preheat the oven to 300°F.

- ❖ Remove from oven and stir in dates and raisins. Allow to cool completely.
- ❖ Store in an airtight place Up to 2 weeks in a jar.
- ❖ Place 1/2 cup of granola in a container for each serving and apply milk.

11) Omelette with vegetables and caramelized onions

Preparation Time: 6 min   **Cooking Time**: 6 min   **Servings: 6**

Ingredients:

- ✓ 1 tablespoon of extra virgin olive oil
- ✓ One small white onion, finely sliced
- ✓ 1/4 teaspoon of brown sugar
- ✓ 1/8 teaspoon crushed black pepper
- ✓ Omelette
- ✓ 2-3 tablespoons of organic olive oil
- ✓ 1 1/2 cups sawn zucchini
- ✓ 1 garlic clove, minced
- ✓ One cup of finely chopped mushrooms
- ✓ 2-3 tablespoons of thinly sliced fresh basil

Ingredients:

- ✓ 1 tablespoon sliced fresh parsley or 1 tablespoon dried parsley
- ✓ Spinach in two cups
- ✓ Four complete eggs
- ✓ Five egg whites
- ✓ 1/2 cup of milk 1%
- ✓ 1/2 cup shredded low-fat pepper jack cheese
- ✓ 1/8 teaspoon sea salt
- ✓ Cracked black pepper
- ✓ Heat the oven to 350 degrees F.
- ❖ Add the zucchini and cook for about a minute. Insert the garlic, and sauté another 2 to 3 minutes before adding the mushrooms, basil, and parsley.
- ❖ Cook vegetables for another minute, sprinkle vegetables with salt and pepper (mushrooms will produce water and are not tan. If you add the salt right away). 8. Comb through, turn off the heat and add the spinach to a large bowl, mix in all the eggs, egg whites, milk, shredded cheese, salt and pepper.
- ❖ Drizzle a 9-inch round cake pan with olive oil spray. Pour in the sautéed components and then the egg mixture.
- ❖ Place the pan on the middle rack of the stove, and bake for 20-25 minutes, or when it comes out clean from a knife implanted in the center.

Directions:

- ❖ To caramelize the onions, heat a medium saucepan to a reasonable temperature.
- ❖ Introduce the oil and when the oil is hot, include the onion, sugar and pepper.
- ❖ Allow the onion to "sweat," pushing it to avoid burning once every moment, before it turns light brown and softened, perhaps ten minutes.
- ❖ Turn off the heat and protect the pan. When you go to serve,
- ❖ You begin by heating a large skillet over medium heat to start the frittata. Then you add the oil.

12) Oatmeal for apples and spices

Preparation Time: 6 min   **Cooking Time**: 6 min   **Servings: 1**

Ingredients:

- ✓ One sweet apple, cut, peeled, such as Gala or Golden Delicious, and cut to 1/2 inch
- ✓ Nuts 2/3 cups water
- ✓ 1/3 cup (rolled) of old oats
- ✓ Pinch of ground cinnamon

Ingredients:

- ✓ Pinch of freshly chopped nutmeg
- ✓ A couple of grains of kosher salt
- ✓ 1/2 cup milk, fat-free, to serve

Directions:

- ❖ Integrate the apples, water, oats, cinnamon, nutmeg and salt in a shallow saucepan.
- ❖ Over medium heat, bring to a boil, lower heat to low, and cap. Simmer for about four minutes before the oats are tender.
- ❖ In a 1-quart microwave-safe dish, mix the apple, water, cinnamon, oats, nutmeg and salt.

- ❖ Use plastic wrap and microwave on high power for about four minutes before oats are tender.
- ❖ Reveal carefully, stir and let stand for 1 minute.
- ❖ In a bowl, move the oatmeal, pour in the milk and serve.

13) Whole wheat strawberry and maple compote pancakes

Preparation Time: 3 min   **Cooking Time**: 6 min   **Servings: 6**

Ingredients:

- ✓ Compote
- ✓ Fresh strawberries, one pound (1 quart) cored and finely chopped 1/4 cup maple syrup
- ✓ Pancakes
- ✓ One cup of whole wheat pasta flour
- ✓ 1/2 cup superfine whole wheat flour
- ✓ Sugar per 1 teaspoon.

Ingredients:

- ✓ 11/2 teaspoon baking powder
- ✓ 1/4 teaspoon. kosher salt.
- ✓ 11/2 cup low-fat milk (1%)
- ✓ 1 huge egg plus 2 big white eggs
- ✓ In a pump sprayer, two teaspoons of canola or corn oil, and more

Directions:

- ❖ Compote: In a medium bowl, combine the strawberries and maple syrup.
- ❖ Leave the strawberries at room temperature to allow the fluids to be released at room temperature. A minimum of 1 hour and up to 4 hours.
- ❖ To make the pancakes: preheat the oven to 200°F. In a medium bowl, mix together the whole wheat dough flour, unbleached flour, sugar, salt and baking powder.
- ❖ Mix the milk, egg and egg whites and the 2 tablespoons of oil. Add the dry ingredients and mix until just combined.

- ❖ Over medium-high heat, heat a grill pan (ideally nonstick). Drizzle it with a little oil.
- ❖ For each pancake, add 1/4 cup of batter to grill pan. Cook until the top is done.
- ❖ The top of each pancake is covered with a bubble for about two minutes. Flip the pancakes over with a large spatula and bake for a few minutes until the undersides are golden brown, about 1 minute longer.
- ❖ On a baking sheet, move pancakes and keep leftover pancakes warm in the oven before preparing.

14) Blueberries and yogurt cornmeal waffles

Preparation Time: 5 min   **Cooking Time**: 10 min   **Servings**: 8

Ingredients:

- ✓ One cup unbleached whole wheat flour
- ✓ One cup of cornmeal that is really yellow
- ✓ Sugar 2 teaspoons
- ✓ 1 1/2 teaspoon baking powder
- ✓ 1/4 teaspoon of kosher salt
- ✓ 1 3/4 cups low-fat milk (1%)

Ingredients:

- ✓ 1 tablespoon unsalted butter, melted
- ✓ 1 tablespoon canola or corn oil, plus more in a pump sprayer,
- ✓ Two main egg whites
- ✓ Two cups regular low-fat yogurt to serve, at room temperature,
- ✓ Two containers of blueberries (6 ounces) (about 2 2/3 cups), at room temperature, to serve.

Directions:

- ❖ Preheat oven to 200°F. Preheat a nonstick waffle iron as per instructions from the maker.
- ❖ in a large bowl, mix together all the flour, cornmeal, sugar, baking powder and salt.
- ❖ Mix milk, melted butter and 1 tablespoon oil in a small bowl Add dry ingredients and stir with a wooden spoon until products are dry.
- ❖ Just lightly mixed with flour strips; should not over mix.
- ❖ Pull egg whites with an electric immersion blender into a separate bowl at high speed just until stiff peaks are reached and not dry.
- ❖ In the batter, bring in the whites. Spray oil onto waffle iron. (Do not use nonstick spray with aerosol.) (Do not use nonstick spray with aerosol.) Pour 1 cup of batter into waffle iron (exact amount depends on scale of waffle iron) cover iron and cook according to manufacturer's instructions before is waffle golden brown.
- ❖ From the iron, cut out the waffle, move to a baking sheet and keep the oven warm when making the remaining waffles.
- ❖ Divide the squares into waffles. Stack 2 waffle squares on a plate for each serving.
- ❖ Top with 1/4 cup yogurt and 1/3 cup blueberries and serve immediately.

15) Banana smoothie berries

Preparation Time: 5 min   **Cooking Time**: 10 min   **Servings:**

Ingredients:

- ✓ 1/2 ripe banana, ideally frozen
- ✓ 1/2 cup fresh or frozen blueberries
- ✓ 1/2 cup low-fat milk (1/%)

Directions:

- ❖ Slice and chop the banana into pieces.

Ingredients:

- ✓ 1/2 cup low-fat yogurt
- ✓ 1/4 teaspoon of vanilla extract
- ✓ 1 tablespoon of amber agave nectar (optional)
- ❖ Blend all products, such as sweetener (if used), when creamy, in a processor.
- ❖ Place in a tall glass and serve immediately.

16) Chocolate and Peanut Butter Smoothie

Preparation Time: 5 min   **Cooking Time**: 10 min   **Servings**: 2

Ingredients:

- ✓ A ripe banana, at least overnight, stored
- ✓ 2/3 cup low-fat milk (1%)
- ✓ 2/3 cup low-fat yogurt
- ✓ Crispy peanut butter 2 tablespoons.

Directions:

- ❖ Slice and chop the banana into pieces.
- ❖ Blend bananas in a blender with milk, yogurt, peanut butter, sugar substitute (if using), cocoa powder and ice cubes.

Ingredients:

- ✓ Two teaspoons of unsweetened cocoa powder
- ✓ One tablespoon of amber agave nectar (optional)
- ✓ Four ice cubes

- ❖ Load into two large glasses and serve immediately.

17) Cabbage and apple smoothie

Preparation Time: 8 min   **Cooking Time**: 10 min   **Servings**: 1

Ingredients:

- ✓ 1 cup kale leaves, well washed, shredded and loose
- ✓ 1/2 cup Jonathan or Gala sweet fruit, cored and coarsely chopped
- ✓ 1/3 cup apple cider vinegar

Directions:

- ❖ In a blender, blend all ingredients until creamy.

Ingredients:

- ✓ 2 tablespoons of sunflower seeds
- ✓ Six ice cubes
- ✓ Eight leaves of healthy mint

- ❖ Sprinkle into a tall glass and serve instantly.

18) Lassi mango

Preparation Time: 15 min   **Cooking Time**: none   **Servings**: 1

Ingredients:

- ✓ One ripe mango, pitted, sliced and coarsely chopped 1/2 cup
- ✓ Smooth without fat
- ✓ yogurt

Directions:

- ❖ Blend the mango cubes, yogurt, milk and ice until smooth.

Ingredients:

- ✓ 1/2 cup fat-free milk
- ✓ Three ice cubes
- ✓ Pinch of ground cardamom (optional)

- ❖ Pour into a long glass. Sprinkle with cardamom, if using. Serve immediately.

19) Papaya and Coconut Breakfast Smoothie

Preparation Time: 11 min   **Cooking Time**: none   **Servings**: 2

Ingredients:

- ✓ One ripe papaya, seed and skin removed and cut into 1-inch chunks
- ✓ A cup of low-fat yogurt
- ✓ One cup of water with coconut (not coconut milk)

Directions:

- ❖ In a processor, puree all materials, such as sweetener (if used).

Ingredients:

- ✓ Two tablespoons of wheat germ
- ✓ 1/2 teaspoon of zero-calorie sweetener (optional)

- ❖ Pour into 2 large glasses and serve.

20) Cappuccino at home

Preparation Time: 10 min   **Cooking Time**: 10 min   **Servings: 2**

Ingredients:

✓   One cup of low-fat (1%) or fat-free milk

Directions:

❖ Heat milk over medium heat in a small saucepan until it steams. (Or heat in a microwave for about 1 minute on high heat).

❖ Meanwhile, bring fresh water to the base of the coffee maker up to the steam nozzle.

❖ To the basket, transfer the coffee beans by screwing it up to the top. Bring to a boil at high temperature and cook until the coffee has stopped splashing under the lid through the longitudinal spout.

Ingredients:

✓   Three tablespoons of ground coffee beans

❖ Remove that from the heat of the temperature.

❖ In a blender, pour in the hot milk and process once sticky.

❖ Divide the coffee into two coffee cups. Pour the same amount of milk from the blender to cover the coffee with the remaining milk, then pour in. Serve hot.

21) Green Tea Ginger

Preparation Time: 5 min   **Cooking Time**: 8 min   **Servings: 1**

Ingredients:

✓   Two quarter-sized strips of fresh, unpeeled ginger
✓   3/4 cup of water

Directions:

❖ In a small skillet, place the ginger and beat the pieces with the edge of a wooden spoon.

❖ Include water and at high temperature, bring to a boil.

Ingredients:

✓   One green tea bag

❖ In a cup, insert a tea bag. With the ginger, pour in the hot water. Allow 2 to 3 minutes for steeping.

❖ Remove the ginger and tea bag, using only a spoon.

❖ Drink warm.

22) Buckwheat crepes

Preparation Time: 5 min   **Cooking Time**: 10 min   **Servings: 6**

Ingredients:

✓   One cup of buckwheat flour
✓   1/3 cup whole wheat flour
✓   One beaten egg

Directions:

❖ Mix and match all the elements in the mixing bowl and beat until you have a consistent batter.

❖ Heat nonstick skillet for three minutes on high heat.

❖ Ladle in a small amount of batter. And straighten the pan in the style of a crepe.

Ingredients:

✓   One cup of skimmed milk
✓   One teaspoon of olive oil
✓   1/2 teaspoon ground cinnamon

❖ For 1 min, cook it and flip it to the other side. Cook it for an extra 30 seconds.

❖ With the leftover batter, repeat the previous procedure.

23) Muffins with carrots

Preparation Time: 5 min   **Cooking Time**: 10 min   **Servings: 5**

Ingredients:

- ✓ 1 1/2 cups whole wheat flour
- ✓ ½ cup stevia
- ✓ 1 tablespoon baking powder
- ✓ ½ teaspoon cinnamon powder
- ✓ ½ tablespoon of cooking soda
- ✓ ¼ cup of natural apple juice
- ✓ Olive oil about ¼ cup

Directions:

- ❖ Combine the flour and stevia in a large bowl, baking powder, baking soda and cinnamon and mix well.
- ❖ Include apple juice, oil, blueberries, carrots, cranberries, ginger and pecans. But very well shaken.

Ingredients:

- ✓ 1 single egg
- ✓ Fresh Blueberries 1 cup
- ✓ Two carrots, grated
- ✓ Ginger 2 tablespoons, brushed
- ✓ ¼ cup chopped pecans
- ✓ Cooking spray

- ❖ Grease a muffin pan with cooking spray, divide the muffin mixture, place in the oven and bake for thirty minutes at 375 degrees Fahrenheit
- ❖ Divide muffins between plates and serve for breakfast. Love!

24) Chia seed breakfast mix

Preparation Time: 8 hours   **Cooking Time**: none   **Servings: 4**

Ingredients:

- ✓ Old fashioned oats with 2 cups
- ✓ Four tablespoons of chia seeds
- ✓ Four tablespoons of coconut sugar

Directions:

- ❖ Integrate oats with chia seeds, sugar, milk, lemon and chia seeds in a cup.

Ingredients:

- ✓ THREE cups of coconut milk
- ✓ 1 teaspoon of lemon zest, minced
- ✓ Blueberries 1 cup
- ❖ Stir in zest and blueberries, divide into cups and keep in refrigerator. For 8 hours.
- ❖ For breakfast, serve. Enjoy!

25) High Energy Porridge

Preparation Time: 15-20 min   **Cooking Time**: 15 min   **Servings: 4**

Ingredients:

- ✓ 200ml whole milk
- ✓ 35g (1¼oz) porridge oats

Directions:

- ❖ In a skillet, combine all ingredients, heat the pan and boil the mixture for about 3-4 minutes.

Ingredients:

- ✓ Optional: add a little cream and syrup or jam for extra energy
- ❖ Or you can cook it for about 1-2 minutes in the microwave, stirring at 30 second intervals.

26) Blueberry and Pineapple Smoothie

Preparation Time: 15 min   **Cooking Time**: None   **Servings: 2**

Ingredients:

- ✓ ½ cup of water
- ✓ ½ apple
- ✓ ½ cup of English cucumber

Directions:

- ❖ In a blender, add the blueberries, cucumber, pineapple, apple and water and combine until thick.

Ingredients:

- ✓ ½ cup of pineapple chunks
- ✓ 1 cup of frozen blueberries

- ❖ Pour smoothie into 2 glasses and enjoy.

27) The Beach Boy Omelette

Preparation Time: 5 min   **Cooking Time**: 5-10 min   **Servings: 1**

Ingredients:

- ✓ 2 sprigs of parsley
- ✓ 1 tablespoon of soy milk
- ✓ 2 egg whites
- ✓ 1 whole egg

Directions:

- ❖ Heat the oil and add the onion and pepper. Sauté for about 2 minutes.
- ❖ Add the browns with the shredded hash and simmer for another 5 minutes.
- ❖ Whip the milk and eggs and place the mixture in a separate omelet tray.

Ingredients:

- ✓ 2 tablespoons of frozen shredded hash browns
- ✓ 2 tablespoons of diced green bell pepper
- ✓ 2 tablespoons of diced onion
- ✓ 1 tablespoon of canola oil
- ❖ Cook until your omelet is firm.
- ❖ Place the hash brown mixture in the center of the omelet and roll the omelet up.
- ❖ Garnish with new parsley to serve.

28) Traditional English breakfast cooked

Preparation Time: 5 min   **Cooking Time**: 5 min   **Servings: 1**

Ingredients:

- ✓ 4 small mushrooms or 1 small tomato, or 2 tablespoons of cooked beans
- ✓ 2 pieces of bacon or 1 sausage (remove fat or opt for low fat if trying to lose weight)

Directions:

- ❖ If you are trying to lose weight, then grilling is the safest way to cook, or you can fry with minimal oil in a non-stick pan or use spray oil.

Ingredients:

- ✓ All the toast you want (though be careful if you're trying to lose weight)
- ✓ 1 egg - as you prefer

- ❖ Then frying in fat can help increase the calories in your breakfast if you need to add weight.

29) Apple and Thai Smoothie

Preparation Time: 5 minutes, plus 30 minutes maceration time   **Cooking Time**: 5 min   **Servings: 2**

Ingredients:

- ✓ 2 cups of ice
- ✓ 1 apple, peeled, pitted and cut into pieces

Directions:

- ❖ Heat rice milk in a large saucepan over medium-low heat for about 5 minutes or until steaming.
- ❖ Remove the milk from the heat and add the infused tea bag.

Ingredients:

- ✓ 1 sachet of chai tea
- ✓ 1 cup unsweetened rice milk
- ❖ Let the milk cool for about 30 minutes in the refrigerator with the sachet, and then remove the sachet, squeezing gently to release all the flavor.
- ❖ In a blender, place the milk, apple and ice and blend until smooth.
- ❖ Pour into 2 glasses and serve.

30) Bagel with egg and salmon

Preparation Time: 10 min   **Cooking Time**: 10 min   **Servings**: 1

Ingredients:

- ✓ 1 oz. cooked salmon
- ✓ 1 large egg
- ✓ 1 slice of tomato
- ✓ 4 pieces of rocket
- ✓ 1 tablespoon of cream cheese

Directions:

- ❖ In a toaster oven or microwave, cut the bagel in half and toast one half.
- ❖ Chop dill leaves, shallots and basil. Mix with the cream cheese.
- ❖ Spread cream cheese mixture over half of the toasted bagel, then top with arugula and tomato slice.

Ingredients:

- ✓ 2 leaves of fresh basil
- ✓ 1/2 teaspoon fresh dill
- ✓ 1 tablespoon shallot
- ✓ 1/2 bagel

- ❖ Heat a skillet, spray with a little nonstick cooking oil spray and scramble the eggs.
- ❖ In the same pan, add the salmon while the egg is cooking.
- ❖ Place the egg and salmon on top of your tomato slices. And enjoy!

31) Apple and onion omelette

Preparation Time: 5 to 10 min   **Cooking Time**: 20 min   **Servings**: 2

Ingredients:

- ✓ 1 tablespoon butter
- ✓ 1/8 teaspoon black pepper
- ✓ 1 tablespoon water
- ✓ 1/4 cup of 1% low-fat milk

Directions:

- ❖ Preheat the oven to about 400° F.
- ❖ Peel and decorate the apple. Slice the apple and onion thinly.
- ❖ Beat eggs in a small bowl with water, milk and pepper; set aside.
- ❖ Melt butter in a medium-sized baking pan over medium-low heat.
- ❖ Add the onion and apple to the skillet and sauté for about 5 to 6 minutes before the onion becomes transparent.

Ingredients:

- ✓ 3 big eggs
- ✓ 3/4 cup of sweet onion
- ✓ 1 large apple
- ✓ 2 tablespoons shredded cheddar cheese
- ❖ In skillet, spread onion and apple mixture equally.
- ❖ Generously pour the egg mixture into the skillet and cook until the sides tend to settle over medium-high heat. Sprinkle the cheddar cheese on top. Move the pan to the oven and bake for about 10-12 minutes, until the center is firmly cooked.
- ❖ Halve the omelet and slide each half onto an individual plate. Serve immediately.

32) Bagel bread pudding

Preparation Time: 15 min   **Cooking Time**: 30 min   **Servings: 2**

Ingredients:
- ✓ 1 teaspoon of cinnamon
- ✓ 1/4 cup sugar
- ✓ 1/4 cup of low-cholesterol egg replacer

Directions:
- ❖ Preheat oven or toaster oven to about 350°F. Drizzle 1 tablespoon of cooking oil on a shallow baking sheet.
- ❖ Divide the bagel and place in a baking dish into small pieces.
- ❖ Mix the egg, sugar, almond milk and cinnamon together and add on top of the bagel pieces.

Ingredients:
- ✓ 1/2 cup of almond milk
- ✓ 1 medium bagel

- ❖ Set aside for a few minutes before the bagels use up the liquid.
- ❖ Bake for about 30 minutes or until the top is golden brown. Serve cold or warm. If needed, add whipped topping.

33) Cinnamon apple bread

Preparation Time: 20 min   **Cooking Time**: 12 min   **Servings: 12**

Ingredients:
- ✓ 1/2 cup of milk
- ✓ 1-1/2 cups all-purpose flour
- ✓ 2 big eggs
- ✓ 2/3 cup of granulated sugar
- ✓ 1-1/2 teaspoon ground cinnamon

Directions:
- ❖ Preheat the oven to about 350° F. Prepare the butter to smooth it out. Grease a 9 x 5-inch loaf pan. Peel and finely chop the apple.
- ❖ In a cup, combine the brown sugar with the cinnamon and set aside.
- ❖ Combine granulated sugar and butter in a standing mixer until smooth.
- ❖ Incorporate eggs and vanilla; continue beating until blended, at a medium pace.
- ❖ Stir in flour and baking powder; begin combining until combined. Add the egg and pour into the batter.

Ingredients:
- ✓ 1/2 cup of packed light brown sugar
- ✓ 2 teaspoons of vanilla extract
- ✓ 1 large apple
- ✓ 1-1/2 teaspoon baking powder
- ✓ 1/2 cup unsalted butter

- ❖ In the baking dish, add half of the prepared batter, and then finish with half of the sliced apples and half of the cinnamon-sugar mixture.
- ❖ Pour over the remaining batter. Stir in the remaining apples and gently dab them with the back of a spoon onto the batter. Cover with remaining cinnamon-sugar mixture and gently dab, again.
- ❖ Bake for 45-55 minutes or until clean, with a toothpick inserted into the center of the loaf. Allow 10 minutes to cool before moving to a cooling rack from the loaf tray.
- ❖ Divide the cooled sandwich into twelve 3/4-inch pieces.

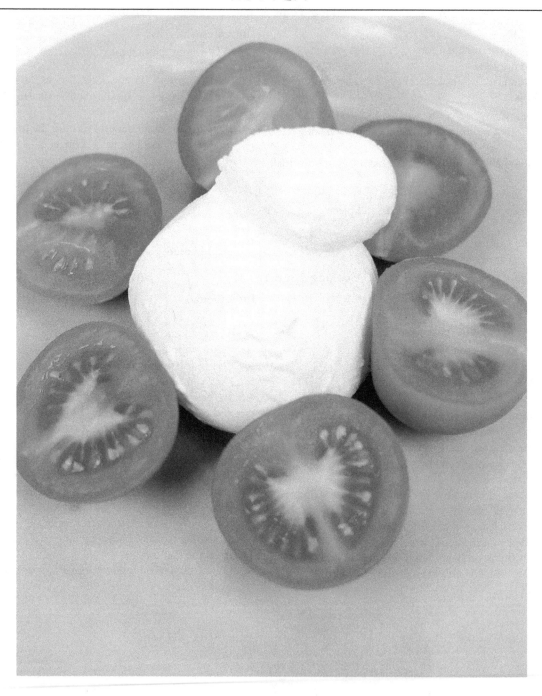

34) Quick pan-fried chicken

Preparation Time: 10 min   **Cooking Time**: 10 min   **Servings: 4**

Ingredients:

- ✓ 2 tablespoons of dried basil
- ✓ 2 spoons of honey
- ✓ 2 tablespoons of balsamic vinegar

Directions:

- ❖ Heat olive oil over medium heat in a skillet. Sprinkle with pepper and toss with chicken.
- ❖ Fry the chicken on both sides for 5 minutes, until golden brown.
- ❖ Add the balsamic vinegar and sauté, turning the chicken to cover, for one minute.

Ingredients:

- ✓ 1/4 teaspoon of black pepper
- ✓ 1 pound boneless, skinless chicken breasts
- ✓ 2 tablespoons of olive oil
- ❖ Apply the basil and honey. Stir and turn to cover the chicken. Cook longer for 1 minute.
- ❖ Mix the sauce in a dish and pour over the chicken.

35) Pilaf rice better than packaged rice

Preparation Time: 10 min   **Cooking Time**: 25 min   **Servings: 6**

Ingredients:

- ✓ 1 tablespoon of chicken broth granules
- ✓ 1 cup parboiled rice, uncooked
- ✓ 2 ounces of vermicelli noodles, uncooked

Directions:

- ❖ Melt 1 tablespoon butter over medium-high heat in a skillet.
- ❖ Divide vermicelli into 2-inch portions and cook until noodles begin to brown, stirring regularly.
- ❖ Substitute the leftover rice and butter. Stir to combine.

Ingredients:

- ✓ 2 cups of water
- ✓ 2 tablespoons unsalted butter
- ✓ 1 tablespoon onion and herb seasoning mix
- ❖ In the skillet, apply the chicken bouillon granules, water and herb seasoning. To mix ingredients, whisk.
- ❖ Cover and bring to a boil. Lower the heat and simmer for 20 minutes. Do not remove the lid.
- ❖ Turn off the heat and prepare for another 5 minutes to stay covered.
- ❖ Flatten and serve with a fork.

36) Pan-fried chicken, green beans and potatoes

Preparation Time: 10 min   **Cooking Time**: 25 to 30 min   **Servings: 4**

Ingredients:

- ✓ 1 tablespoon dry mix of Italian seasoning
- ✓ 4 tablespoons unsalted butter
- ✓ 10 ounces of frozen cut green beans

Directions:

- ❖ Preheat the oven to about 400° F.
- ❖ Peel the potatoes and cut them up. Place in a large pot of water and bring to a boil for 10 minutes. Drain, add fresh water, bring to a boil and cook potatoes for about 10 minutes, until tender. Drain and return. If you don't need a low potassium strategy, skip this step. Break only the unpeeled potatoes into chunks.

Ingredients:

- ✓ 16 ounces of thin, raw chicken strips
- ✓ 3 cups of red potatoes
- ❖ Use cooking spray to spray a 9 x 13-inch baking dish. Place 1/3 of the baking sheet on top of the chicken strips. Arrange about 1/3 of the baking sheet with the green beans and the last 1/3 of the baking sheet with the potatoes.
- ❖ Melt the butter and pour the green beans, chicken and potatoes over the entire plate. Sprinkle the dry Italian seasoning mixture over the entire plate.
- ❖ Bake for about 20-30 minutes.

37) Pan-fried Brussels sprouts and pears

Preparation Time: 15 min   **Cooking Time**: 15 min   **Servings: 4**

Ingredients:
- ✓ 1 tablespoon of balsamic vinegar glaze
- ✓ 2 tablespoons of olive oil

Directions:
- ❖ Preheat the oven to about 400° F.
- ❖ Remove outer leaves from Brussels sprouts and split in half. Core and cut into 1/2-inch cubes with the unpeeled pears.
- ❖ In a cup, place 1 teaspoon of olive oil. Add Brussels sprouts and toss with oil to cover.
- ❖ Move Brussels sprouts to a 9 x 13-inch baking dish and spread over half of the dish in a continuous layer. For 12 minutes, roast.

Ingredients:
- ✓ 2 medium fresh pears
- ✓ 2-1/2 cups Brussels sprouts
- ❖ Place the remaining teaspoon in the bowl with the olive oil. Stir in the diced pears and toss with the oil until covered.
- ❖ Remove the sprouts from the oven and add the pears to the other half of the dish. Roast for another 12 minutes, or until the pears are soft.
- ❖ In a serving dish, toss the Brussels sprouts and pears together. Drizzle with 1 teaspoon balsamic vinegar glaze and serve.

38) Roasted cauliflower with rosemary

Preparation Time: 15 min   **Cooking Time**: 30 min   **Servings: 9**

Ingredients:
- ✓ 1/4 teaspoon of black pepper
- ✓ 1/4 teaspoon salt
- ✓ 1-1/2 tablespoon olive oil

Directions:
- ❖ Preheat the oven to about 450° F.
- ❖ Break cauliflower florets into chunks. Rosemary chops.
- ❖ Place cauliflower with remaining ingredients in a large dish.

Ingredients:
- ✓ 1 tablespoon fresh rosemary
- ✓ 6 cups of cauliflower florets

- ❖ Spread the seasoned cauliflower on an ungreased baking sheet.
- ❖ For 15 minutes, roast; remove from oven and stir.
- ❖ Continue roasting for 10 minutes or until cauliflower is gently browned and soft.

39) Roasted Brussels sprouts, carrots and apples

Preparation Time: 15 min.   **Cooking Time**: 30 to 40 min   **Servings: 8**

Ingredients:
- ✓ 1/4 teaspoon salt
- ✓ 1/2 teaspoon of nutmeg
- ✓ 1 teaspoon of cinnamon
- ✓ 2 tablespoons of maple syrup

Directions:
- ❖ Preheat oven to about 375° F. Use nonstick cooking spray to spray a baking sheet.
- ❖ Cut Brussels sprouts and split in half. Peel and cut carrots into 1-inch pieces. Core and split apples into 1/2-inch pieces.
- ❖ Place the sprouts, carrots, and Brussels apple pieces in a large dish.

Ingredients:
- ✓ 1/4 cup olive oil
- ✓ 2 medium apples
- ✓ 3 large carrots
- ✓ 20 medium Brussels sprouts
- ❖ Combine the olive oil, maple syrup and spices in a shallow bowl. Stir to combine.
- ❖ Pour vegetable mixture with sauce and toss to coat. On baking sheet, place ingredients. Sprinkle with 1/4 teaspoon salt if necessary.
- ❖ Cook until carrots are fork tender and Brussels sprouts begin to soften 30-40 minutes.

40) Grilled steak with vegetables in vinaigrette

Preparation Time: 15 min   **Cooking Time**: 20 min   **Servings: 8**

Ingredients:

- ✓ 1/4 cup fresh flat leaf parsley
- ✓ 1 garlic clove
- ✓ 2 tablespoons of balsamic vinegar
- ✓ 6 tablespoons of extra virgin olive oil
- ✓ 2 medium peppers

Directions:

- ❖ Heat the grill to a medium-high temperature.
- ❖ Add 1/4 teaspoon salt and 1/2 teaspoon pepper to steak.
- ❖ for medium cooking, grill steak until perfectly cooked, 4 to 5 minutes per hand.
- ❖ Move the steak to a cutting board and let it rest for at least 5 minutes before cutting.
- ❖ Cut the eggplant into four 1/2-inch thick circles when the steak is frying. Cut the bell paper into quarters and remove the seed.

Ingredients:

- ✓ 1 medium eggplant
- ✓ 1 teaspoon of black pepper
- ✓ 1/2 teaspoon salt
- ✓ 1 pound of beef steak

- ❖ Using 3 tablespoons gasoline, wash all sides of eggplant and peppers. Stir in remaining 1/4 teaspoon salt and 1/2 teaspoon pepper for seasoning.
- ❖ Grill vegetables until soft, 4 to 5 minutes on both sides.
- ❖ Remove one garlic clove and chop parsley. Combine the remaining milk, vinegar, garlic and parsley in a small bowl to create a vinaigrette sauce.
- ❖ Divide the steak and vegetables among four dinner plates.
- ❖ Pour sauce over vegetables or eat on the side.

41) Mushrooms Florentine style

Preparation Time: 10 minutes   **Cooking Time**: 10 minutes   **Servings: 4**

Ingredients:

- ✓ 5 ounces of whole wheat pasta
- ✓ 1/4 cup low-sodium chicken broth
- ✓ 1 cup mushrooms, sliced

Directions:

- ❖ Cook the pasta according to the box guide.
- ❖ Then pour the saucepan with the olive oil and heat it up.
- ❖ Add the Italian seasonings and mushrooms. Mix well with the mushrooms and simmer for 10 minutes.

Ingredients:

- ✓ 1/4 cup soy milk
- ✓ 1 teaspoon of olive oil
- ✓ 1/2 teaspoon of Italian seasonings
- ❖ Then add the chicken broth and soy milk.
- ❖ Stir the mixture well and add the cooked pasta. Cook over low heat for 5 minutes.

42) Bean hummus

Preparation Time: 10 minutes   **Cooking Time**: 40 minutes   **Servings: 4**

Ingredients:

- ✓   1 cup of chickpeas, soaked
- ✓   6 cups of water
- ✓   1 tablespoon of tahini paste
- ✓   2 garlic cloves,

Directions:

- ❖   Pour the water into the pot, add the chickpeas and close the lid.
- ❖   Cook chickpeas for 40 minutes on low heat or until soft.
- ❖   After this, transfer the cooked chickpeas to the food processor.

Ingredients:

- ✓   ¼ cup olive oil
- ✓   ¼ cup of lemon juice
- ✓   1 teaspoon of harissa

- ❖   Add the olive oil, lemon juice, harissa, garlic cloves and tahini paste.
- ❖   Blend the hummus until smooth.

43) Hasselback eggplants

Preparation Time: 15 minutes   **Cooking Time**: 20 minutes   **Servings: 2**

Ingredients:

- ✓   2 eggplants, cut
- ✓   2 tomatoes, sliced
- ✓   1 tablespoon of low-fat yogurt

Directions:

- ❖   Create cuts in the Hasselback pattern in the eggplant.
- ❖   Then rub the curry powder over the vegetables and line them up with the sliced tomatoes.

Ingredients:

- ✓   1 teaspoon of curry powder
- ✓   1 teaspoon of olive oil

- ❖   Drizzle olive oil and yogurt over eggplant and cover in foil (place each Hasselback eggplant separately).
- ❖   For 25 minutes, cook vegetables at 375F.

44) Vegetarian Kebab

Preparation Time: 10 minutes   **Cooking Time**: 10 minutes   **Servings: 4**

Ingredients:

- ✓   2 tablespoons of balsamic vinegar
- ✓   1 tablespoon of olive oil
- ✓   1 teaspoon of dried parsley
- ✓   2 tablespoons water

Directions:

- ❖   Break onions and sweet peppers into medium-sized squares.
- ❖   Then break up the zucchini.
- ❖   Thread the skewers with all the vegetables.
- ❖   After that, mix the olive oil, dried parsley, water and balsamic vinegar in a small dish.

Ingredients:

- ✓   2 sweet peppers
- ✓   2 red onions, peeled
- ✓   2 zucchini, cut

- ❖   Drizzle the vegetable skewers with the olive oil mixture and transfer to a grill preheated to 390F.
- ❖   Cook skewers on both sides for 3 minutes or until vegetables are light brown.

45) White bean stew

Preparation Time: 10 minutes   **Cooking Time**: 50 minutes   **Servings: 4**

Ingredients:

- ✓ 1 cup white beans, soaked
- ✓ 1 cup low-sodium chicken broth
- ✓ 1 cup zucchini, chopped
- ✓ 1 teaspoon of tomato paste
- ✓ 1 tablespoon avocado oil

Directions:

- ❖ Heat avocado oil in saucepan, add zucchini and roast for 5 minutes.
- ❖ After this, add the white beans, chicken broth, tomato paste, water, peppercorns, ground black pepper and ground nutmeg.

Ingredients:

- ✓ 4 cups of water
- ✓ ½ teaspoon of peppercorns
- ✓ ½ teaspoon of ground black pepper
- ✓ ¼ teaspoon ground nutmeg

- ❖ Close the lid and cook the stew for 50 minutes over low heat.

46) Vegetarian Lasagna

Preparation Time: 10 minutes   **Cooking Time**: 30 minutes   **Servings: 4**

Ingredients:

- ✓ 1 cup carrot, diced
- ✓ ½ cup bell bell pepper, diced
- ✓ 1 cup spinach, chopped
- ✓ 1 tablespoon of olive oil
- ✓ 1 teaspoon of chili powder

Directions:

- ❖ Place the carrot, bell bell pepper and spinach in the saucepan.
- ❖ Add the olive oil and chili powder and mix the vegetables well.
- ❖ Cook them for 5 minutes.

Ingredients:

- ✓ 1 cup tomatoes, chopped
- ✓ 4 ounces of low-fat cottage cheese
- ✓ 1 eggplant, sliced
- ✓ 1 cup low-sodium chicken broth

- ❖ After that, make the sliced eggplant layer in the casserole mold and cover it with the vegetable mixture.
- ❖ Add the tomatoes and ricotta cheese.
- ❖ Bake the lasagna for 30 minutes at 375F.

47) Carrot cakes

Preparation Time: 10 minutes   **Cooking Time**: 5 minutes   **Servings: 4**

Ingredients:

- ✓ 1 cup carrot, grated
- ✓ 1 tablespoon of semolina
- ✓ 1 egg, beaten

Directions:

- ❖ In mixing bowl, mix grated carrot, semolina, egg and Italian seasonings.
- ❖ Heat the sesame oil in the skillet.

Ingredients:

- ✓ 1 teaspoon of Italian seasonings
- ✓ 1 tablespoon of sesame oil

- ❖ Make the carrot cakes with the help of 2 spoons and place them in the pan.
- ❖ Roast the cakes for 4 minutes per side.

48) Vegan Chili

Preparation Time: 10 minutes   **Cooking Time**: 25 minutes   **Servings: 4**

Ingredients:

- ✓ ½ cup of bulgur
- ✓ 1 cup tomatoes, chopped
- ✓ 1 hot pepper, chopped
- ✓ 1 cup red beans, cooked

Ingredients:

- ✓ 2 cups low-sodium chicken broth
- ✓ 1 teaspoon of tomato paste
- ✓ ½ cup celery stalk, chopped

Directions:

❖ Place all ingredients in large saucepan and mix well.

❖ Close the lid and cook the chili for 25 minutes over medium-low heat.

49) **Aromatic whole wheat spaghetti**

Preparation Time: 5 minutes   **Cooking Time**: 10 minutes   **Servings: 4**

Ingredients:

✓ 1 teaspoon of dried basil
✓ ¼ cup soy milk
✓ 6 ounces of whole wheat spaghetti

Directions:

❖ Bring water to a boil, add spaghetti and cook for 8-10 minutes.

❖ Meanwhile, bring the soy milk to a boil.

Ingredients:

✓ 2 cups of water
✓ 1 teaspoon ground nutmeg

❖ Drain cooked noodles and stir in soy milk, nutmeg powder and dried basil.

❖ Mix in the flour well.

50) **Chopped tomatoes**

Preparation Time: 5 minutes   **Cooking Time**: 10 minutes   **Servings: 4**

Ingredients:

✓ 2 cups plum tomatoes, coarsely chopped
✓ ½ cup onion, diced
✓ ½ teaspoon garlic, diced

Directions:

❖ In a saucepan, melt the canola oil.

❖ Add the onion and red pepper. For 5 minutes, prepare the vegetables.

❖ From time to time, stir them.

Ingredients:

✓ 1 teaspoon of Italian seasonings
✓ 1 teaspoon of canola oil
✓ 1 hot pepper, chopped

❖ Attach the onions, garlic and Italian seasonings after this.

❖ Cover the lid and cook the food for 10 minutes.

51) Baked Falafel

Preparation Time: 10 minutes   **Cooking Time**: 25 minutes   **Servings: 4**

Ingredients:

✓ 2 cups of chickpeas, cooked
✓ 1 yellow onion, diced
✓ 3 tablespoons of olive oil
✓ 1 cup fresh parsley, chopped

Directions:

❖ In food processor, place all ingredients and blend until smooth.

❖ At 375F, preheat the oven.

❖ Then, with baking paper, cover the baking sheet.

Ingredients:

✓ 1 teaspoon of ground cumin
✓ ½ teaspoon of coriander
✓ 2 garlic cloves, diced

❖ Create balls from the chickpea mixture and gently press them into falafel shape.

❖ Place the falafels in the baking dish and bake for 25 minutes in the oven.

52) **Paella**

Preparation Time: 10 minutes   **Cooking Time**: 25 minutes   **Servings: 10**

Ingredients:

- ✓ 1 teaspoon of dry saffron
- ✓ 1 cup short-grain rice
- ✓ 1 tablespoon of olive oil
- ✓ 2 cups of water
- ✓ 1 teaspoon of chili flakes

Directions:

- ❖ In the saucepan, add the water. Include the rice and simmer for fifteen minutes.
- ❖ Meanwhile, load the skillet with olive oil.
- ❖ Add the dried saffron, chili flakes, bell bell pepper and onion.

Ingredients:

- ✓ 6 ounces of artichoke hearts, chopped
- ✓ ½ cup green peas
- ✓ 1 onion, sliced
- ✓ 1 cup bell bell pepper, sliced

- ❖ For 5 minutes, roast the vegetables.
- ❖ Apply them to the rice that has been cooked.
- ❖ Then add the artichoke hearts and green peas. Stir the paella well and simmer for 10 minutes.

53) Mushroom cakes

Preparation Time: 15 minutes　　**Cooking Time**: 10 minutes　　**Servings: 4**

Ingredients:

- ✓ 2 cups mushrooms, chopped
- ✓ 3 garlic cloves, minced
- ✓ 1 tablespoon of dried dill
- ✓ 1 egg, beaten

Directions:

- ❖ In food processor, grind mushrooms.
- ❖ Combine the garlic, dill, egg, chili powder and flour.
- ❖ Blend for 10 seconds with the combination.

Ingredients:

- ✓ ¼ cup rice, cooked
- ✓ 1 tablespoon of sesame oil
- ✓ 1 teaspoon of chili powder

- ❖ Heat the sesame oil for 1 minute afterwards.
- ❖ Form medium-sized mushroom cakes and place them in the hot sesame oil.
- ❖ Cook the mushroom cakes over medium heat for 5 minutes on each side.

54) Glazed eggplant rings

Preparation Time: 10 minutes　　**Cooking Time**: 10 minutes　　**Servings: 2**

Ingredients:

- ✓ 3 eggplants, sliced
- ✓ 1 tablespoon liquid honey
- ✓ 1 teaspoon chopped ginger
- ✓ 2 tablespoons of lemon juice

Directions:

- ❖ Use ground cilantro to scrub eggplant.
- ❖ Then heat the avocado oil for 1 minute in a skillet.
- ❖ Add the sliced eggplant and assemble in a layer when the oil is hot.
- ❖ Cook vegetables on one side for 1 minute.

Ingredients:

- ✓ 3 tablespoons of avocado oil
- ✓ ½ teaspoon of ground coriander
- ✓ 3 tablespoons of water

- ❖ Place eggplant on a plate.
- ❖ Then coat the pan with chopped ginger, liquid sugar, lemon juice and water.
- ❖ Bring to a boil and add the eggplant that has been cooked.
- ❖ Coat the vegetables well in the sweet liquid and simmer for another 2 minutes.

55) Sweet potato balls

Preparation Time: 15 minutes   **Cooking Time**: 10-15 minutes   **Servings: 4**

Ingredients:

- ✓ 1 cup sweet potato, mashed, cooked
- ✓ 1 tablespoon fresh cilantro, chopped
- ✓ 1 egg, beaten
- ✓ 3 tablespoons ground oatmeal

Directions:

- ❖ In bowl, mix mashed sweet potato, fresh cilantro, egg, ground oatmeal, paprika and turmeric.
- ❖ Stir the mixture until smooth and make balls.

Ingredients:

- ✓ 1 teaspoon ground paprika
- ✓ ½ teaspoon ground turmeric
- ✓ 2 tablespoons of coconut oil

- ❖ Heat the coconut oil in the saucepan.
- ❖ When the coconut oil is hot, add the sweet potato balls.
- ❖ Cook them until they are golden brown.

56) Chickpea curry

Preparation Time: 10 minutes   **Cooking Time**: 5 minutes   **Servings: 4**

Ingredients:

- ✓ 1 ½ cup chickpeas, boiled
- ✓ 1 teaspoon of curry powder
- ✓ ½ teaspoon of gram masala
- ✓ 1 cup spinach, chopped

Directions:

- ❖ Heat the coconut oil in the saucepan.
- ❖ Add the curry powder, gram masala, tomato paste and soy milk.
- ❖ Blend the mixture until smooth and bring it to a boil.

Ingredients:

- ✓ 1 teaspoon of coconut oil
- ✓ ¼ cup soy milk
- ✓ 1 tablespoon of tomato paste
- ✓ ½ cup of water
- ❖ Add water, spinach and chickpeas.
- ❖ Stir in the flour and close the lid.
- ❖ Cook for 5 minutes over medium heat.

57) Bowl of quinoa

Preparation Time: 15 minutes   **Cooking Time**: 15 minutes   **Servings: 4**

Ingredients:

- ✓ 1 cup of quinoa
- ✓ 2 cups of water
- ✓ 1 cup of tomatoes, diced
- ✓ 1 cup sweet bell pepper, diced

Directions:

- ❖ Mix the water and quinoa together, and then simmer for 15 minutes. Then remove it from the sun and let it sit for 10 minutes to rest.
- ❖ Move the cooked quinoa to a large plate.

Ingredients:

- ✓ ½ cup rice, cooked
- ✓ 1 tablespoon of lemon juice
- ✓ ½ teaspoon lemon zest, grated
- ✓ 1 tablespoon of olive oil
- ❖ Add the tomatoes, peppers, corn, lemon juice, olive oil and lemon zest.
- ❖ Mix the mixture well in the serving bowls and pass.

58) Vegan meatloaf

Preparation Time: 10 minutes   **Cooking Time**: 8 minutes   **Servings: 2**

Ingredients:

- ✓ 1 cup chickpeas, cooked
- ✓ 1 onion, diced
- ✓ 1 tablespoon ground flaxseed
- ✓ ½ teaspoon of chili flakes

Directions:

- ❖ Heat the coconut oil in the saucepan.
- ❖ Add the carrot, onion, and celery stalk. Cook the vegetables for 8 minutes or until soft.
- ❖ Then add the chickpeas, chili flakes and ground flax seeds.

Ingredients:

- ✓ 1 tablespoon of coconut oil
- ✓ ½ cup carrot, diced
- ✓ ½ cup celery stalk, chopped
- ✓ 1 tablespoon of tomato paste
- ❖ Blend the mixture until smooth using an immersion blender.
- ❖ Then, line the loaf mold with baking paper and transfer the mixed mixture inside.
- ❖ Flatten well and spread with tomato paste.
- ❖ Bake the meatloaf in the preheated 365F oven for 20 minutes.

59) Loaded potato skins

Preparation Time: 15 minutes   **Cooking Time**: 30 minutes   **Servings: 4**

Ingredients:

- ✓ 6 potatoes
- ✓ 1 teaspoon of ground black pepper
- ✓ 2 tablespoons of olive oil

Directions:

- ❖ Preheat the oven to 400F.
- ❖ Pierce potatoes with the help of the knife 2-3 times and bake for 30 minutes or until vegetables are tender.
- ❖ After that, cut the baked potatoes in half and scoop out the potato flesh into the bowl.

Ingredients:

- ✓ ½ teaspoon of minced garlic
- ✓ ¼ cup soy milk

- ❖ Drizzle the potato halves with olive oil and ground black pepper and return to the oven. Bake for 15 minutes or until light brown.
- ❖ Meanwhile, mash the harvested potato meat and mix it with the soy milk and minced garlic.
- ❖ Fill the cooked potato halves with the mashed potato mixture.

60) Vegan meat pie

Preparation Time: 10 minutes   **Cooking Time**: 25 minutes   **Servings: 4**

Ingredients:

- ✓ ½ cup quinoa, cooked
- ✓ ½ cup of tomato puree
- ✓ ½ cup carrot, diced
- ✓ 1 shallot, chopped

Directions:

- ❖ In a saucepan, place the carrots, scallions, and mushrooms.
- ❖ Add the coconut oil and cook the vegetables until tender but not foamy, 10 minutes or until tender.
- ❖ Then combine the cooked vegetables with the tomato puree and chili powder.

Ingredients:

- ✓ 1 tablespoon of coconut oil
- ✓ ½ cup potato, cooked, mashed
- ✓ 1 teaspoon of chili powder
- ✓ ½ cup mushrooms, sliced
- ❖ Shift the mixture and flatten it well into the casserole shape.
- ❖ Comb the vegetables with the mashed potatoes after this. Cover the shepherd's pie with aluminum foil and bake for 25 minutes in the preheated 375F oven.

61) Cauliflower steaks

Preparation Time: 15 minutes   **Cooking Time**: 25 minutes   **Servings: 4**

Ingredients:

- ✓ 1 lb cauliflower head
- ✓ 1 teaspoon ground turmeric
- ✓ ½ teaspoon of cayenne pepper

Directions:

- ❖ Slice head of cauliflower and rub with ground turmeric, cayenne pepper and garlic powder.
- ❖ Then line the baking sheet with baking paper and place the cauliflower steaks inside.

Ingredients:

- ✓ 2 tablespoons of olive oil
- ✓ ½ teaspoon of garlic powder

- ❖ Drizzle with olive oil and bake at 375F for 25 minutes or until vegetable steaks are tender.

62) Delicious vegetarian quesadillas

Preparation Time: 10 minutes   **Cooking Time**: 3-7 minutes   **Servings: 3**

Ingredients:

- ✓ One cup of refried black beans
- ✓ 1/2 bell red bell pepper, chopped
- ✓ Cilantro 4 pieces, chopped
- ✓ 1/2 cup corn
- ✓ One cup of cheddar, low fat, shredded

Directions:

- ❖ Divide one-quarter of the tortillas with the black beans, red bell bell pepper, two tablespoons of cilantro, corn, carrot, jalapeno and cheese and combine with the remaining tortillas.
- ❖ Over medium-high heat, heat a skillet, insert a quesadilla, cook on one side for three minutes, flip, cook on the other for another minute and move to a tray.

Ingredients:

- ✓ Six whole wheat tortillas
- ✓ One slice of carrot, shredded
- ✓ One small jalapeno bell pepper, diced
- ✓ 1 cup of yogurt, fat-free
- ✓ Juice of 1/2 lime
- ❖ for the rest of the quesadillas, repeat.
- ❖ Combine two tablespoons of the cilantro with the yogurt and lime juice in a bowl. Mix well and serve alongside the quesadillas.

63) Chicken Wraps

Preparation Time: 10 minutes   **Cooking Time**: 5 minutes   **Servings: 4**

Ingredients:

- ✓ Chicken breast, 8 ounces, cubed
- ✓ 1/2 cup celery, chopped
- ✓ 2/3 of a cup of mandarin oranges, sliced
- ✓ 1/4 cup chopped onion
- ✓ A splash of olive oil

Directions:

- ❖ Over high heat with oil, add chicken cubes, cook on each side for 5 minutes, and move to a bowl.

Ingredients:

- ✓ Mayonnaise 2 tablespoons
- ✓ 1/4 teaspoon crushed garlic
- ✓ A sprinkle of black pepper
- ✓ Four whole grain tortillas
- ✓ Four leaves of lettuce
- ❖ On each tortilla divide the meat, also divide the celery, grapes, cabbage, mayonnaise, garlic powder, black pepper and lettuce leaves, roll up and serve for lunch.

64) Black bean meatballs

Preparation Time: 10 minutes   **Cooking Time**: 5 minutes   **Servings: 4**

Ingredients:

- ✓ Two slices of whole wheat pizza, broken
- ✓ Cilantro 3 teaspoons, chopped
- ✓ Two garlic cloves, diced
- ✓ 15 ounces of dried black beans, no salt added, washed and rinsed
- ✓ Six ounces of dried and chopped chipotle peppers
- ✓ 1 cumin paste, field

Directions:

- ❖ In your bowl, place the crust, wipe well, and mash crumbs into a cup.
- ❖ Integrate in this mixture with cilantro, garlic, black beans, chipotle peppers, cumin and egg, mix well and form 4 patties.

Ingredients:

- ✓ 1 single egg
- ✓ Kitchen spray
- ✓ 1/2 avocado peeled, pitted and mashed
- ✓ 1 tablespoon of lime juice
- ✓ 1 tomato plum, chopped

- ❖ Heat a skillet over medium-high heat, grease with cooking spray, add the bean patties, and cook on each side for five minutes and transfer to plates.
- ❖ Mix avocado with tomato and lime juice in a cup, mix well, add to meatballs and serve for lunch.

65) Lunch rice bowls

Preparation Time: 10 minutes   **Cooking Time**: 5 minutes   **Servings: 2**

Ingredients:

- ✓ 1 tablespoon of olive oil
- ✓ One cup mixed peppers, onions, zucchini and cabbage, chopped
- ✓ 1 cup chicken meat, fried and shredded
- ✓ 1 cup cooked brown rice

Directions:

- ❖ Over medium-high heat, heat a skillet with oil, add mixed vegetables, swirl and simmer for five minutes.

Ingredients:

- ✓ Three tablespoons of sauce
- ✓ Low-fat cheddar for 2 teaspoons, sliced
- ✓ Two tablespoons of low-fat sour cream

- ❖ Divide the chicken meat and rice into two containers, insert the mixed vegetables and add the sauce, cheese and sour cream to each.
- ❖ Serve during the lunch hour.

66) Lunch Salmon salad

Preparation Time: 10 minutes   **Cooking Time**: 5 minutes   **Servings: 3**

Ingredients:

- ✓ 1 cup canned salmon, flaked
- ✓ 1 tablespoon of lemon juice
- ✓ Three tablespoons of fat-free yogurt
- ✓ Two tablespoons of chopped red bell pepper
- ✓ 1 tablespoon capers, drained and chopped

Directions:

- ❖ Integrate the lemon juice, yogurt, bell bell pepper, capers, onion, dill and black pepper with the salmon in a bowl and mix well.

Ingredients:

- ✓ One tablespoon of chopped red onion
- ✓ 1 teaspoon dill, chopped
- ✓ A sprinkle of black pepper
- ✓ Three slices of wholemeal bread

- ❖ Spread it on any slice of bread and have it for lunch.

67) Stuffed mushrooms caps

Preparation Time: 10 minutes   **Cooking Time**: 15 minutes   **Servings: 2**

Ingredients:

- ✓ Two caps of Portobello mushrooms
- ✓ Pesto 2 tablespoons.

Directions:

- ❖ In each mushroom cap, divide the pesto, tomato and mozzarella, arrange them on a rimmed baking sheet, place in the oven and bake for fifteen minutes at 400 degrees Fahrenheit

Ingredients:

- ✓ Two tomatoes, cut
- ✓ 1/4 cup mozzarella cheese, low-fat, sliced
- ❖ For lunch, serve.

68) Lunch Tuna salad

Preparation Time: 10 minutes   **Cooking Time**: None   **Servings: 3**

Ingredients:

- ✓ Five ounces of dried tuna soaked in water
- ✓ 1 tablespoon of red vinegar
- ✓ Olive oil, 1 tablespoon.
- ✓ 1/4 cup chopped green onions

Directions:

- ❖ Mix the tuna with the vinegar, oil, arugula, pasta, green onions and black pepper in a bowl. Stir.

Ingredients:

- ✓ Arugula two cups
- ✓ 1 tablespoon of grated low-fat Parmesan cheese
- ✓ A sprinkle of black pepper
- ✓ Two ounces of whole wheat pasta, cooked
- ❖ Divide among three baking sheets, sprinkle parmesan cheese on top and serve for lunch.

69) Shrimp rolls for lunch

Preparation Time: 10 minutes   **Cooking Time**: None   **Servings: 4**

Ingredients:

- ✓ 12 sheets of rice paper, soaked only for a few seconds in hot water and drained
- ✓ Sliced 1 cup cilantro
- ✓ 12 basil leaves
- ✓ 12 baby lettuce leaves

Directions:

- ❖ On a work surface, arrange all rice papers, begin dividing cilantro, bay leaves, small lettuce leaves, cucumber, carrots and shrimp, wrap, seal edges and serve for lunch.

Ingredients:

- ✓ A small sliced cucumber
- ✓ One cup of chopped carrots
- ✓ 20 ounces of shrimp, cooked, shelled and uncooked

70) Turkey sandwich

Preparation Time: 10 minutes   **Cooking Time**: 3 minutes   **Servings: 2**

Ingredients:
- ✓ Two slices of wholemeal bread
- ✓ Mustard 2 teaspoons
- ✓ Smoked turkey Two cubes

Ingredients:
- ✓ 1 pear, cut and cored
- ✓ 1/4 cup mozzarella cheese, low-fat, sliced

Directions:
- ❖ Pour mustard on each slice of bread, divide turkey slices on one slice of bread, insert pear slices and mozzarella cheese, cover with the other slice of bread, add three minutes to the grill of the hot oven, cut sand in half and serve.

71) Vegetarian soup

Preparation Time: 10 minutes   **Cooking Time**: 5 minutes   **Servings: 6**

Ingredients:
- ✓ Two teaspoons of olive oil
- ✓ 1 and 1/2 cup carrots, shredded
- ✓ Six garlic cloves, minced
- ✓ 1 cup chopped yellow onion
- ✓ 1 cup diced celery

Ingredients:
- ✓ Low sodium chicken broth per 32 ounces
- ✓ Four cups of water
- ✓ 1 and 1/2 cup whole wheat pasta
- ✓ Sawn 2 tablespoons of parsley
- ✓ 1/4 cup low-fat grated Parmesan cheese
- ❖ Add the onion, water and pasta, stir, bring to a boil and cook for another eight minutes over medium heat.

Directions:
- ❖ Over medium-high heat, heat pots with oil adds garlic, stir and simmer for 1 minute.
- ❖ Insert the onion, celery and carrot, stir and roast for 7 minutes.
- ❖ Divide among cups, cover and serve each with parsley and Parmesan cheese.

72) Lunch salad with melon and avocado

Preparation Time: 10 minutes   **Cooking Time**: None   **Servings: 4**

Ingredients:
- ✓ Stevia for 2 tablespoons
- ✓ Two tablespoons of red vinegar
- ✓ Chopped 2 teaspoons of spices,
- ✓ A sprinkle of black pepper
- ✓ One avocado peeled, pitted and diced

Ingredients:
- ✓ Four cups of baby spinach
- ✓ 1/2 thin melon, peeled and diced
- ✓ 1 1/2 cups sliced strawberries
- ✓ 2 teaspoons of sesame, toasted seeds

Directions:
- ❖ Integrate the avocado with the lettuce, melon and strawberries in a salad bowl and toss.

- ❖ Include stevia with vinegar, mint and black pepper in another pan, shake, add to salad, toss, top with sesame seeds and serve.

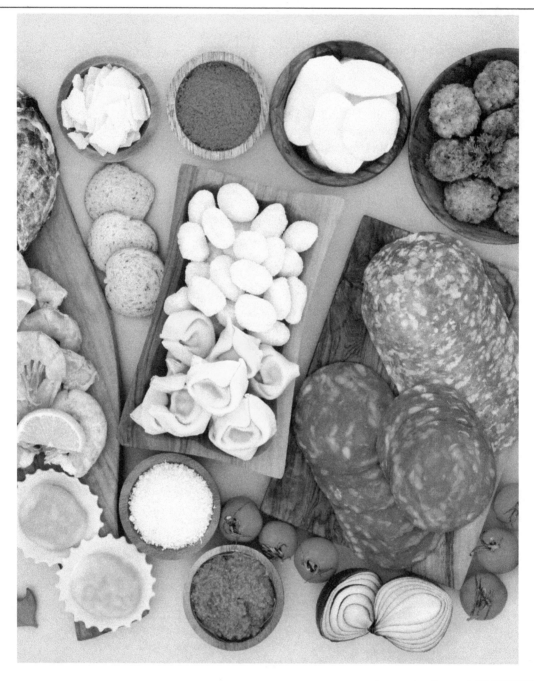

73) Soft goulash

Preparation Time: 10 minutes   **Cooking Time**: 50 minutes   **Servings: 4**

Ingredients:

- ✓ 1 pound of beef tenderloin, minced
- ✓ 2 garlic cloves, peeled
- ✓ ½ teaspoon ground clove

Ingredients:

- ✓ ¼ teaspoon ground cardamom
- ✓ 2 onions, diced
- ✓ 1 cup of water
- ❖ Add all remaining ingredients and close the lid.
- ❖ Cook the goulash over medium heat for 50 minutes.

Directions:

- ❖ Rub the beef tenderloin with the ground clove and cardamom.
- ❖ Place the meat in the casserole dish.

74) Steak chunks with cayenne pepper

Preparation Time: 10 minutes   **Cooking Time**: 24 minutes   **Servings: 4**

Ingredients:

- ✓ 1 lb beefsteak
- ✓ 1 teaspoon of cayenne pepper

Ingredients:

- ✓ 1 teaspoon of olive oil

- ❖ Then drizzle the meat with olive oil and place it in the tray in one layer.
- ❖ Bake the meat at 360F for 12 minutes per side.

Directions:

- ❖ Rub the flank steak with cayenne pepper and cut into bites.

75) Beef brussels sprouts

Preparation Time: 5 minutes   **Cooking Time**: 40 minutes   **Servings: 4**

Ingredients:

- ✓ 1 cup Brussels sprouts, chopped
- ✓ 12 ounces of beef sirloin, minced
- ✓ 1 cup of water

Ingredients:

- ✓ 1 teaspoon of peppercorns
- ✓ 1 teaspoon ground paprika
- ✓ 1 teaspoon of dried basil
- ❖ Close the lid and cook the beef over medium heat for 40 minutes or until the beef is tender.

Directions:

- ❖ Place all ingredients in the saucepan and mix well.

76) Beef with cauliflower

Preparation Time: 10 minutes   **Cooking Time**: 50 minutes   **Servings: 4**

Ingredients:

- ✓ 1 cup cauliflower, chopped
- ✓ 12 ounces of beef tenderloin, minced
- ✓ 1 clove of garlic, diced

Ingredients:

- ✓ 1 cup of water
- ✓ 1 teaspoon of dried thyme

- ❖ Add the cauliflower and close the lid.
- ❖ Cook beef over medium heat for 50 minutes. Stir occasionally.

Directions:

- ❖ Mix beef with dried thyme and diced garlic.
- ❖ Place the beef in the casserole dish and add the water.

77) Beef Stroganoff without mushrooms

Preparation Time: 10 minutes **Cooking Time**: 30 minutes **Servings: 4**

Ingredients:

- ✓ 12 ounces of sirloin steak, cut into strips
- ✓ 1 tablespoon of olive oil
- ✓ 1 cup of water
- ✓ 1 teaspoon of white flour

Ingredients:

- ✓ 1 teaspoon of minced garlic
- ✓ ¼ cup of rice milk
- ✓ 1 onion, sliced

Directions:

- ❖ Pour the olive oil into the casserole dish and preheat it.
- ❖ Add the beefsteak and minced garlic.
- ❖ Roast the meat for 2 minutes per side.
- ❖ After this, add the onion, water and rice milk.
- ❖ Stir the mixture and bring it to a boil. Simmer the meat for 10 minutes.
- ❖ Then add the white flour and mix in the flour until smooth.
- ❖ Close the lid and cook the meat for another 5 minutes.

78) Beef tips

Preparation Time: 10 minutes **Cooking Time**: 25 minutes **Servings: 4**

Ingredients:

- ✓ 14 ounces of beef loin, minced
- ✓ 1 oz shallot, chopped
- ✓ 1 clove of garlic, diced

Ingredients:

- ✓ ¼ teaspoon ground ginger
- ✓ 1 tablespoon of olive oil
- ✓ ½ cup of water
- ❖ Close the lid and cook the beef over medium heat for 20 minutes.
- ❖ When the meat is tender, it is cooked.

Directions:

- ❖ Roast the beef loin with olive oil for 2 minutes per side.
- ❖ Then add all the remaining ingredients and mix gently.

79) Pulled Beef

Preparation Time: 10 minutes **Cooking Time**: 65 minutes **Servings: 4**

Ingredients:

- ✓ Loin of beef 1 pound
- ✓ 1 teaspoon of peppercorns

Ingredients:

- ✓ 1 teaspoon of dried basil
- ✓ 4 cups of water
- ❖ Close the lid and cook the meat over medium heat for 65 minutes.
- ❖ Then cool the meat to room temperature and remove it from the liquid.
- ❖ Shred the meat with the help of a fork and add ¼ cup of the remaining liquid.

Directions:

- ❖ Pour the water into the saucepan.
- ❖ Add the dried basil, peppercorns and water.
- ❖ Add the beef loin.

80) Italian Spices Beef

Preparation Time: 10 minutes   **Cooking Time**: 50 minutes   **Servings: 4**

Ingredients:

✓   1 tablespoon of Italian seasonings

Directions:

❖   Rub the beef loin with Italian seasonings and drizzle with canola oil.

Ingredients:

✓   Loin of beef 1 pound
✓   1 teaspoon of canola oil

❖   Wrap beef in foil and bake at 360F for 50 minutes.

81) Shredded beef

Preparation Time: 10 minutes   **Cooking Time**: 65 minutes   **Servings: 4**

Ingredients:

✓   1 lb beef tenderloin
✓   1 cup of water

Directions:

❖   Place the beef tenderloin in the casserole dish.
❖   Add the water, red pepper and ground nutmeg.

Ingredients:

✓   1 hot pepper
✓   ¼ teaspoon ground nutmeg

❖   Close the lid and cook the meat over medium heat for 60 minutes.
❖   Remove the meat from the liquid and shred it.

82) Tender veal chops

Preparation Time: 10 minutes   **Cooking Time**: 30 minutes   **Servings: 4**

Ingredients:

✓   ½ cup of rice milk
✓   1 lb veal chops

Directions:

❖   Sprinkle the veal chops with the ground nutmeg.
❖   Then preheat the canola oil well.

Ingredients:

✓   1 teaspoon ground nutmeg
✓   1 tablespoon of canola oil

❖   Place the veal chops in the oil and roast for 3 minutes per side.
❖   After this, add the rice milk and close the lid.
❖   Cook veal chops over medium heat for 20 minutes.

83) Onions stuffed with beef

Preparation Time: 10 minutes   **Cooking Time**: 40 minutes   **Servings: 4**

Ingredients:

✓   4 onions, peeled
✓   6 ounces of beef tenderloin, minced
✓   ¼ teaspoon minced garlic

Directions:

❖   Make holes in the onion.
❖   Then mix the beef with the minced garlic and ground clove.

Ingredients:

✓   ¼ teaspoon of ground clove
✓   ½ cup of water

❖   Fill the onions with the meat mixture and place them in the baking dish in one layer.
❖   Add the water and transfer the pan to the oven.
❖   Bake the meal at 360F for 40 minutes.

84) Beef and vegetable bowl

Preparation Time: 20 minutes   **Cooking Time**: 30 minutes   **Servings: 4**

Ingredients:

- ✓ 12 ounces of beef loin, minced
- ✓ 2 peppers, chopped
- ✓ 1 cup okra, chopped

Directions:

- ❖ Pour the water into the saucepan.
- ❖ Add the beef loin, peppers, okra, chili powder and dried thyme.

Ingredients:

- ✓ 1 cup of water
- ✓ 1 teaspoon of chili powder
- ✓ ½ teaspoon of dried thyme
- ❖ Close the lid and cook the meal over medium heat for 30 minutes.
- ❖ Then remove the meal from the heat and let it sit for 10 minutes to rest.
- ❖ Place meal in bowls.

85) Baked Beef Tray

Preparation Time: 10 minutes   **Cooking Time**: 40 minutes   **Servings: 4**

Ingredients:

- ✓ 1 cup okra, sliced
- ✓ 16 ounces of beef tenderloin, cut into strips

Directions:

- ❖ Mix the beef tenderloin with the ground cilantro and place in the tray.

Ingredients:

- ✓ ¼ cup of water
- ✓ 1 teaspoon of ground coriander
- ❖ Add the okra and water.
- ❖ Transfer the tray to the oven and bake at 360F for 40 minutes

86) Beef with cumin

Preparation Time: 10 minutes   **Cooking Time**: 30 minutes   **Servings: 4**

Ingredients:

- ✓ 12 ounces beef tenderloin, coarsely chopped
- ✓ 1 tablespoon of cumin seeds

Directions:

- ❖ Mix beef tenderloin with cumin seeds, olive oil and soy milk.

Ingredients:

- ✓ 1 tablespoon of olive oil
- ✓ ¼ cup soy milk
- ❖ Transfer the meat mixture to the casserole dish and close the lid.
- ❖ Cook the meat over medium heat for 30 minutes.

87) Beef with cilantro

Preparation Time: 10 minutes   **Cooking Time**: 55 minutes   **Servings: 4**

Ingredients:

- ✓ 1 tablespoon of dried coriander

Directions:

- ❖ Pour the water into the saucepan.

Ingredients:

- ✓ 1 cup of water
- ✓ 10 ounces of beef loin
- ❖ Add the beef loin and dried cilantro.
- ❖ Close the lid and cook the meat over medium heat for 55 minutes.

88) Beef curry

Preparation Time: 10 minutes   **Cooking Time**: 40 minutes   **Servings: 4**

Ingredients:

✓ 1 cup of soy milk
✓ 1 onion, diced

Directions:

❖ Pour the soy milk into the saucepan.
❖ Add the diced onion and curry powder. Stir the mixture until smooth.

Ingredients:

✓ 1 tablespoon curry powder
✓ 12 ounces of beef tenderloin, minced

❖ Add the beef tenderloin and close the lid.
❖ Cook meat over medium heat for 40 minutes or until meat is tender.

89) Beef with thyme

Preparation Time: 10 minutes   **Cooking Time**: 65 minutes   **Servings: 4**

Ingredients:

✓ 1 tablespoon of dried thyme

Directions:

❖ Rub the beef tenderloin with dried thyme.

Ingredients:

✓ 1 tablespoon of olive oil
✓ 1 lb beef tenderloin

❖ Drizzle the meat with olive oil and wrap in foil.
❖ Bake the meat at 360F for 65 minutes.

90) Beef rolls

Preparation Time: 10 minutes   **Cooking Time**: 45 minutes   **Servings: 4**

Ingredients:

✓ 8 ounces of beef loin
✓ 2 peppers, cut into strips

Directions:

❖ Slice the beef loin into fillets.
❖ Then place the peppers on the fillets.
❖ Sprinkle with ground nutmeg and roll up.

Ingredients:

✓ 1 teaspoon ground nutmeg
✓ 1 cup of water

❖ Secure the rolls with toothpicks and place them in the pot.
❖ Add the water and close the lid.
❖ Cook beef rolls for 45 minutes over medium heat.

91) Cajun beef chunks

Preparation Time: 5 minutes   **Cooking Time**: 20 minutes   **Servings: 4**

Ingredients:

✓ 1 tablespoon Cajun seasonings

Directions:

❖ Mix beef with oil and Cajun seasonings.

Ingredients:

✓ 1 pound of beef tenderloin, minced
✓ 1 teaspoon of olive oil

❖ Then place the beef chunks in the skillet and roast for 5 minutes per side.
❖ Close the lid and cook the meat over medium heat for another 10 minutes.

92) Easy baked beef

Preparation Time: 10 minutes   **Cooking Time**: 60 minutes   **Servings: 4**

Ingredients:

- ✓ 1 carrot, diced
- ✓ 1 clove of garlic, diced
- ✓ ½ cup of water

Directions:

- ❖ Place the beef tenderloin in the pot.

Ingredients:

- ✓ 1 teaspoon of dried rosemary
- ✓ 1 lb beef tenderloin

- ❖ Add all remaining ingredients and close the lid.
- ❖ Transfer the pan to the oven and bake at 365F for 60 minutes

93) Beef cutlets with sage

Preparation Time: 10 minutes   **Cooking Time**: 8 minutes   **Servings: 4**

Ingredients:

- ✓ 1 tablespoon of dried sage
- ✓ 1 pound of beef cutlets

Directions:

- ❖ Rub beef cutlets with ground cumin and dried sage.

Ingredients:

- ✓ ½ teaspoon of ground cumin

- ❖ Then preheat the grill to 390F.
- ❖ Place the cutlets in the grill and cook for 4 minutes per side.

94) Slices of grilled steak

Preparation Time: 10 minutes   **Cooking Time**: 10 minutes   **Servings: 4**

Ingredients:

- ✓ 1 teaspoon of dried oregano
- ✓ 1 tablespoon of olive oil

Directions:

- ❖ Mix beef slices with dried oregano, olive oil and chopped onion.

Ingredients:

- ✓ 1 lb. beef steak, coarsely chopped
- ✓ 1 teaspoon chopped onion

- ❖ Preheat the grill to 400F.
- ❖ Place the beef slices in the grill and cook for 5 minutes per side.

95) Aromatic beef saute

Preparation Time: 10 minutes   **Cooking Time**: 40 minutes   **Servings: 4**

Ingredients:

- ✓ 1 apple, chopped
- ✓ 10 ounces of beef loin, minced
- ✓ 1 clove of garlic, diced

Directions:

- ❖ Place all ingredients in the saucepan and stir gently.

Ingredients:

- ✓ ½ cup broccoli, chopped
- ✓ 1 cup of water
- ✓ 1 teaspoon ground turmeric
- ❖ Close the lid and cook the saute over medium heat for 40 minutes.

96) Burger Casserole

Preparation Time: 20 minutes   **Cooking Time**: 50 minutes   **Servings: 8**

Ingredients:

- ✓ 10 ounces of beef loin, minced
- ✓ 1 teaspoon of dried parsley
- ✓ ½ teaspoon of dried basil

Directions:

- ❖ Mix beef loin with dried parsley, basil and garlic powder.
- ❖ Make small burgers with the meat mixture and place them in the casserole dish.

Ingredients:

- ✓ 1 teaspoon garlic powder
- ✓ 1 cup of cabbage, shredded
- ✓ ½ cup of rice milk
- ❖ Top the burgers with the cabbage and rice milk.
- ❖ Then cover the casserole dish with aluminum foil.
- ❖ Bake the casserole at 360F for 50 minutes.

97) Tender marinated beef

Preparation Time: 25 minutes   **Cooking Time**: 45 minutes   **Servings: 4**

Ingredients:

- ✓ 3 tablespoons of lime juice
- ✓ 1 tablespoon of olive oil
- ✓ 1 teaspoon ground cardamom
- ✓ ¼ teaspoon ground coriander

Directions:

- ❖ Mix lime juice with water, olive oil, ground cardamom, chili powder and ground cilantro.

Ingredients:

- ✓ ½ teaspoon of chili powder
- ✓ ¼ cup of water
- ✓ 1 lb beef tenderloin

- ❖ Place the meat in the liquid and let it marinate for 25 minutes.
- ❖ Then transfer the meat to the tray.
- ❖ Bake the meat at 360F for 45 minutes.

98) Beef meatballs with chili

Preparation Time: 15 minutes   **Cooking Time**: 45 minutes   **Servings: 4**

Ingredients:

- ✓ 1 hot pepper, chopped
- ✓ 1 teaspoon chopped garlic, diced

Directions:

- ❖ Mix the chili with the minced garlic and beef tenderloin.
- ❖ Make small patties with the meat mixture.

Ingredients:

- ✓ 10 ounces of beef tenderloin, minced
- ✓ ¼ cup of water
- ❖ Place the meatballs in the tray in one layer. Add the water.
- ❖ Transfer the tray with the meatballs to the oven and bake at 365F for 45 minutes.

99) Tender boiled beef

Preparation Time: 15 minutes   **Cooking Time**: 70 minutes   **Servings: 4**

Ingredients:
- ✓ 1 teaspoon ground turmeric
- ✓ 1 teaspoon of cinnamon
- ✓ 2 cups of water

Directions:
- ❖ Place all ingredients in the saucepan and close the lid.

Ingredients:
- ✓ ½ hot pepper
- ✓ 12 ounces of beef loin

- ❖ Cook the meal over medium heat for 70 minutes.
- ❖ Then slice the cooked beef into portions and sprinkle with the remaining liquid.

100)   Chicken with cumin

Preparation Time: 10 minutes   **Cooking Time**: 30 minutes   **Servings: 4**

Ingredients:
- ✓ 1 pound chicken breast, skinless, boneless, chopped
- ✓ 1 tablespoon ground cumin

Directions:
- ❖ Mix the chicken breast with the ground cumin and olive oil.

Ingredients:
- ✓ 1 teaspoon of olive oil

- ❖ Place chicken in tray and flatten into a layer.
- ❖ Bake the chicken for 30 minutes at 360F.

101)   Chicken with thyme

Preparation Time: 10 minutes   **Cooking Time**: 30 minutes   **Servings: 4**

Ingredients:
- ✓ 1 pound chicken breast, skinless, boneless, chopped
- ✓ 1 tablespoon of canola oil

Directions:
- ❖ Mix chicken breast with canola oil, dried thyme and soy milk.

Ingredients:
- ✓ 1 teaspoon of dried thyme
- ✓ 1 tablespoon of soy milk

- ❖ Place the chicken in the tray and gently flatten it.
- ❖ Transfer the tray to the oven and bake at 360F for 35 minutes

102)   Chicken with cayenne pepper

Preparation Time: 10 minutes   **Cooking Time**: 30 minutes   **Servings: 4**

Ingredients:
- ✓ 1 teaspoon of cayenne pepper
- ✓ 1 cup of water

Directions:
- ❖ Pour the water into the saucepan.
- ❖ Add the cayenne pepper and bay leaf.

Ingredients:
- ✓ 1 pound of chicken breast, skinless and boneless
- ✓ 1 bay leaf

- ❖ Add the chicken breast and close the lid.
- ❖ Simmer the chicken for 30 minutes over medium heat.

103) Chicken with oregano

Preparation Time: 10 minutes   **Cooking Time**: 10 minutes   **Servings: 4**

Ingredients:
- ✓ 1 lb. chicken fillet, cut into slices
- ✓ 1 tablespoon of dried oregano

Ingredients:
- ✓ 1 tablespoon of olive oil

Directions:
- ❖ Mix sliced chicken with dried oregano and drizzle with olive oil.
- ❖ Preheat the pan well.

- ❖ Place the chicken slices in the pan on one layer and cook for 3 minutes per side.

104) Chicken curry

Preparation Time: 10 minutes   **Cooking Time**: 25 minutes   **Servings: 8**

Ingredients:
- ✓ 1 teaspoon of curry paste
- ✓ 1 cup of soy milk

Ingredients:
- ✓ 1 teaspoon of ground cumin
- ✓ 2 pounds of chicken breast, skinless and boneless

Directions:
- ❖ Mix the curry paste with the soy milk and pour the liquid into the saucepan.
- ❖ Add the ground cumin and chicken breast.

- ❖ Close the lid and cook the chicken over medium heat for 25 minutes.
- ❖ Serve the chicken with the curry paste sauce.

105) Tarragon chicken

Preparation Time: 10 minutes   **Cooking Time**: 10 minutes   **Servings: 5**

Ingredients:
- ✓ 2 pounds chicken breast, skinless, boneless, chopped
- ✓ 1 tablespoon of dried tarragon

Ingredients:
- ✓ 1 tablespoon of canola oil

Directions:
- ❖ Mix chicken breast with dried tarragon and drizzle with canola oil.
- ❖ Preheat the pan well.

- ❖ Place the chicken in the hot skillet. Flatten the chicken pieces into a layer.
- ❖ Roast them for 4 minutes per side over medium-low heat.

106) Chicken with cumin seeds

Preparation Time: 10 minutes   **Cooking Time**: 13 minutes   **Servings: 7**

Ingredients:
- ✓ 1 tablespoon of canola oil
- ✓ 1 tablespoon of cumin seeds

Ingredients:
- ✓ 1 tablespoon of lime juice
- ✓ 2 pounds of chicken fillet, minced

Directions:
- ❖ Pour the canola oil into the pan.
- ❖ Add the chicken fillet and sprinkle with cumin seeds and lime juice.

- ❖ Gently stir the chicken and close the lid.
- ❖ Bake for 10 minutes.
- ❖ Then stir the chicken again and cook for another 3 minutes.

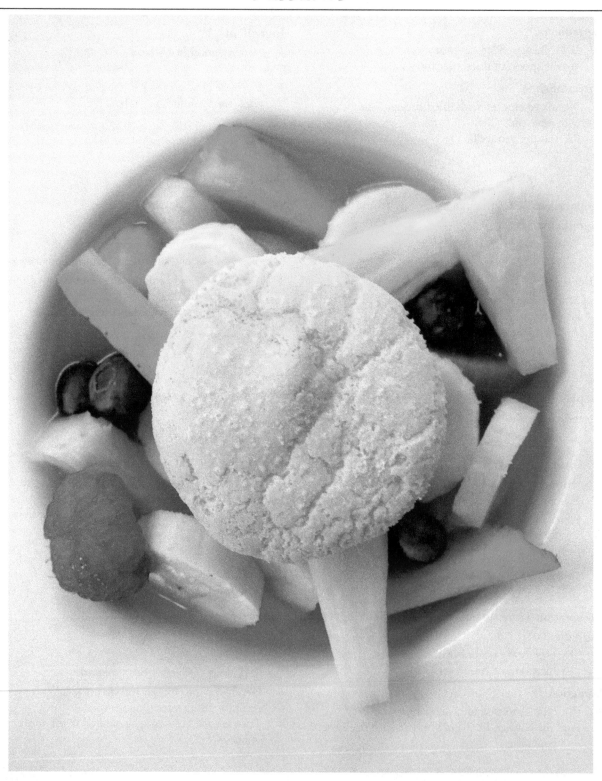

107)   Honey bread pudding

Preparation Time: 15-20 minutes   **Cooking Time**: 40-45 minutes   **Servings: 4**

Ingredients:

- ✓ 6 cups of white bread cubes
- ✓ 1 teaspoon of pure vanilla extract
- ✓ ¼ cup of honey

Directions:

- ❖ Lightly oil a buttered 8-by-8-inch baking dish; set aside.
- ❖ Whisk together the rice milk, eggs, egg whites, sugar and vanilla in a medium bowl.
- ❖ Add the bread cubes and stir until covered with the bread.

Ingredients:

- ✓ 2 large egg whites
- ✓ 2 eggs
- ✓ 1½ cups plain rice milk
- ❖ Move the mixture and cover with plastic wrap in the baking dish.
- ❖ Keep the dish in the refrigerator for a minimum of 3 hours.
- ❖ Preheat the oven to 325°F.
- ❖ Remove the plastic wrap from the pan and bake the pudding for 35-40 minutes, or until a knife inserted in the middle comes out clean and golden brown.
- ❖ Serve hot.

108)   Vanilla Couscous Pudding

Preparation Time: 15-20 minutes   **Cooking Time**: 20 minutes   **Servings: 4**

Ingredients:

- ✓ 1 cup of couscous
- ✓ ¼ teaspoon ground cinnamon
- ✓ ½ cup of honey

Directions:

- ❖ In a large saucepan, combine the water, rice milk and vanilla seeds over medium-low heat.
- ❖ Bring the milk to a gentle boil, reduce the heat to low and let the milk simmer for about 10 minutes to allow the vanilla flavor to enter the milk.
- ❖ Remove the saucepan from the heat.

Ingredients:

- ✓ 1 vanilla pod, separated
- ✓ ½ cup of water
- ✓ 1½ cups plain rice milk
- ❖ Pull out the vanilla pod and remove the seeds from the pod into the hot milk with the tip of a sharp knife.
- ❖ Stir in the cinnamon and sugar.
- ❖ Cover the dish, stir the couscous and let it sit for about 10 minutes.
- ❖ Using a fork, fluff the couscous before eating.

109) Victoria Sponge Cake

Preparation Time: 10 minutes   **Cooking Time**: 35 minutes   **Servings: 4**

Ingredients:

- ✓ 50ml heavy cream
- ✓ A splash of milk (if necessary)
- ✓ 250g (9oz) of self-raising flour
- ✓ 4 medium eggs

Ingredients:

- ✓ 250g (9oz) caster sugar
- ✓ 250g (9oz) unsalted butter, well softened
- ✓ About 5 tablespoons of raspberry jam (add more or less for your favorite flavor)

Directions:

- ❖ Grease two shallow 8-inch cake pans and then line them with baking paper for baking. Preheat the oven to 180°C (160° F) / 350°s F / Gas 4.
- ❖ In a large bowl, include the melted butter and sugar and whisk until very pale and fluffy. This is likely to take about 5-10 minutes. This can be achieved in a standalone mixer, if needed.
- ❖ Apply one egg and one giant spoonful of flour to the mixture and beat again. Until all the eggs are included, repeat this process. Sift out excess flour and then use a large metal spoon to fold over the mixture.

- ❖ Add a splash of milk if the dough doesn't have a droopy consistency (i.e., it slides off a spoon quickly).
- ❖ Spread the mixture between the two pans, smooth the surface and bake for 25 minutes.
- ❖ They should sandwich together until the cakes have been boiled and cooled. Whip the heavy cream until soft peaks form. Spread the jelly on one of the cakes and then spread the whipped cream on top of the jam. Place on top of the second cake and sift in the powdered sugar for decoration.

110) Raspberry Brule

Preparation Time: 15-20 minutes   **Cooking Time**: 1 minutes   **Servings: 4**

Ingredients:

- ✓ 1 cup fresh raspberries
- ✓ ¼ teaspoon ground cinnamon
- ✓ ¼ cup of brown sugar, divided

Ingredients:

- ✓ ½ cup plain cream cheese, room temperature
- ✓ ½ cup light sour cream

Directions:

- ❖ Preheat the baking oven.
- ❖ Beat the heavy cream, cream cheese, 2 teaspoons brown sugar and cinnamon together in a small bowl for about 4 minutes or until very smooth and fluffy.
- ❖ Divide raspberries evenly among four ramekins (4 ounces).

- ❖ Spoon the cream cheese combination over the berries and smooth the tops.
- ❖ Store ramekins until ready to eat dessert in the refrigerator, sealed.
- ❖ On each ramekin, sprinkle 1/2 tablespoon brown sugar evenly.
- ❖ Place the ramekins on a baking sheet until the sugar is caramelized and golden brown, and bake them 4 inches from the heating element.
- ❖ Remove from microwave. Let them rest for 1 minute and serve rules

111) Cherry shortbread

Preparation Time: 20 minutes   **Cooking Time**: 40 minutes   **Servings: 4**

Ingredients:

- ✓ 180g (6oz) plain flour
- ✓ 55g (2oz) of caster sugar, plus extra to finish off

Directions:

- ❖ Heat your oven to about 190°C (170°C fan)/375°F/gas 5.
- ❖ Together, beat the butter and sugar until creamy.
- ❖ To make a smooth dough, whisk in the flour.
- ❖ Apply (if using) cherries and gently stir to blend.

Ingredients:

- ✓ 125g (4oz) unsalted butter
- ✓ Optional: 2 tablespoons of glace cherries - chopped
- ❖ Turn on a work surface and gently roll out until the dough is 1 cm/1⁄2 inch deep.
- ❖ Break it into fingers or rolls and place on a baking sheet. Sprinkle with granulated sugar and chill for 20 minutes in the freezer.
- ❖ Bake for 15-20 minutes in the oven or until golden brown and pale. Set aside on a wire rack to cool.

112) Sweet cinnamon custard

Preparation Time: 20 minutes   **Cooking Time**: 1 hour   **Servings: 6**

Ingredients:

- ✓ 1⁄2 teaspoon ground cinnamon
- ✓ 1 teaspoon of pure vanilla extract
- ✓ 1⁄4 cup granulated sugar
- ✓ 4 eggs

Directions:

- ❖ Preheat the oven to about 325°F.
- ❖ Gently grease six ramekins (4 ounces) and place in baking dish; set aside.
- ❖ Whisk together the eggs, rice milk, vanilla, sugar and cinnamon in a large bowl until you have a very creamy paste.
- ❖ In a pitcher, pour the liquid through a fine sieve.
- ❖ Evenly distribute the custard mixture among the ramekins.

Ingredients:

- ✓ 1⁄2 cups plain rice milk
- ✓ Unsalted butter to grease the ramekins.
- ✓ Cinnamon sticks, for garnish (optional)
- ❖ Rinse the pan with hot water until the water comes halfway up the sides of the ramekins. Be careful not to get water into the ramekins.
- ❖ Bake until the creams are set and a knife inserted into the middle of one of the creams comes out clean, or about 1 hour.
- ❖ Remove the baked creams from the oven and remove the ramekins from the bath.
- ❖ Chill for 1 hour on wire racks and then move the creams to the refrigerator to chill for another hour.
- ❖ Garnish each cream, if necessary, with a cinnamon stick.

113)   Cooled lemon cake

Preparation Time: 5-10 minutes   **Cooking Time:** 45 minutes   **Servings: 4**

Ingredients:

- ✓ 2 cups sugar, powdered variety
- ✓ ¼ cup of lemon juice
- ✓ 1 cup of water

Directions:

- ❖ Preheat the oven to approximately 350° F.
- ❖ Grease a 13' by 9' by 2' baking dish and sift in flour.
- ❖ In a bowl, place the cake mix and combine the applesauce, beaten eggs, and water. You should blend for 30 seconds on low and then switch to medium and blend for another 2 minutes with your food processor.
- ❖ Place flour in the pan and bake until cooked (when inserted, a toothpick comes out clean), about 40 minutes.

Ingredients:

- ✓ 3 eggs
- ✓ ½ cup applesauce, unsweetened
- ✓ 1 box (18 ½ oz.) of a yellow cake mix
- ❖ Cool the cake, then leave it in the pan
- ❖ Combine the lemon juice and powdered sugar until completely mixed.
- ❖ Make slits, each 1/2 inch apart, in the top of the cake.
- ❖ Spoon the lemon glaze over the end, letting it drip into the holes
- ❖ The entire top of the cake would finally be sealed.
- ❖ Relax and work long hours and enjoy

114)   Lemon cheesecake

Preparation Time: 15 minutes   **Cooking Time:**   **Servings: 4**

Ingredients:

For the base
- ✓ 100g (3½oz) soft unsalted butter
- ✓ 200g (7oz) digestive cookies

Directions:

- ❖ Process the cookies in the mixer until they are fine crumbs, then add the butter through the spout in small pieces while the processor is still working. You can end up with a similar quality to wet dough.
- ❖ Butter a jar and firmly push the base mixture into the rim of the jar and place in the refrigerator to set.
- ❖ Beat the cream until it is thickened enough to almost hold its shape, but not quite yet. To save time, use an electronic whisk if you have one.

Ingredients:

For the dressing
- ✓ 1 single dish of cream (or whipping cream, a small dish)
- ✓ 1 packet of cream cheese (a standard packet usually around 200-300 g)
- ✓ Juice of 1 lemon
- ✓ 250g of icing sugar (sifted)
- ❖ In the cream cheese packet, beat until the mixture is smooth.
- ❖ Apply lemon juice and sifted powdered sugar and beat again until strong and thick.
- ❖ Place the topping on the base and spread it out. Return the pan to the refrigerator before the topping has formed. As preferred, include berries.

115)   Baked peaches with cream cheese

Preparation Time: 10 minutes   **Cooking Time**: 15 minutes   **Servings: 4**

Ingredients:

- ✓   1 cup plain cream cheese, room temperature
- ✓   ½ cup crushed meringue cookies (here)
- ✓   ¼ teaspoon ground cinnamon

Directions:

- ❖   Preheat the oven to about 350°F.
- ❖   Cover parchment paper with a baking sheet; set aside.
- ❖   Mix the meringue cookies, cream cheese, cinnamon and nutmeg in a shallow dish.

Ingredients:

- ✓   Pinch of ground nutmeg
- ✓   8 canned peach halves in juice
- ✓   2 spoons of honey
- ❖   Spoon the cream cheese mixture generously over the halves of the cavity peaches.
- ❖   Place peaches on baking sheet and bake until fruit is soft and cheese is melted, or about 15 minutes.
- ❖   Transfer peaches to plates, 2 per individual, from baking dish and drizzle with honey before eating.

116)   Blueberry Peach Crunch

Preparation Time: 15 minutes   **Cooking Time**: 45 minutes   **Servings: 10**

Ingredients:

- ✓   ½ cup unsalted butter
- ✓   ¾ cup packed brown sugar
- ✓   ¾ cup white flour
- ✓   1 tablespoon freshly squeezed lemon juice

Directions:

- ❖   Preheat the oven to approximately 375°F.
- ❖   Stone the peaches and thinly divide them into 3/4-inch strips.
- ❖   "Spray oil on a baking sheet 12" by 9".
- ❖   Arrange the peach slices and blueberries evenly around the base of the dish

Ingredients:

- ✓   ¼ cup of sugar
- ✓   1 cup fresh blueberries
- ✓   7 medium peaches

- ❖   Sprinkle the fruit with lemon juice and honey.
- ❖   In a bowl, mix brown sugar and flour and butter until crumbly.
- ❖   Sprinkle the crumble combination evenly over the berries.
- ❖   Bake for about 45 minutes until the fruit has softened and the crumble is golden brown.
- ❖   Serve hot.

117) Apple Crumble

Preparation Time: 15-20 minutes　　**Cooking Time**: 40-45 minutes　　**Servings: 4**

Ingredients:

For your crumble
- ✓ Butter nut for greasing
- ✓ 200g (7oz) unsalted butter, diced at room temperature
- ✓ 175g (6oz) sugar
- ✓ 300g plain flour, a pinch of sifted salt

Directions:

- ❖ Preheat the oven to about 180 degrees C (160 degrees Fan)/350 degrees F/Gas 4.
- ❖ In a large bowl, place the flour and sugar and combine well. Rub many pieces of butter over the flour mixture at a time. Until the mixture resembles breadcrumbs, continue rubbing.

Ingredients:

For your stuffing
- ✓ 1 pinch of ground cinnamon
- ✓ 1 tablespoon plain flour
- ✓ 50g (2oz) sugar
- ✓ Peeled 450g (1lb) apples, coreless and cut into 1cm/½in pieces
- ❖ In a large bowl, place the fruit and sprinkle in the flour, sugar and cinnamon. Mix well and be careful not to tear the fruit.
- ❖ Butter a 24cm/9-inch baking dish. Spread the fruit mixture on the bottom, then scatter the crumble mix over the top.
- ❖ For 45-50 minutes, bake until crumble is golden brown and fruit mixture is bubbly.

118) Pavlov with peaches

Preparation Time: 30 min plus 1 hour cooling time　　**Cooking Time**: None　　**Servings: 8**

Ingredients:

- ✓ 2 cups canned peaches drained in juice
- ✓ ½ teaspoon of pure vanilla extract
- ✓ 1 cup superfine sugar

Directions:

- ❖ Preheat the oven to about 225°F.
- ❖ Cover parchment paper with a baking sheet; set aside.
- ❖ Beat egg whites in a large bowl for about 1 minute or until soft peaks develop.
- ❖ Beat in the cream of tartar.
- ❖ Add the sugar until the egg whites are very firm and glossy, 1 tablespoon at a time. Do not over beat the eggs.
- ❖ Now whisk in the vanilla.
- ❖ Spread the meringue evenly on the baking sheet, so that you have 8 circles.

Ingredients:

- ✓ ½ teaspoon of cream of tartar
- ✓ 4 large egg whites, at room temperature

- ❖ In the center of each circle, use the back of the spoon to make an indentation.
- ❖ For about 1 hour, bake the meringues or until a light brown crust forms.
- ❖ Turn off the oven and let the meringues rest overnight, still in the oven.
- ❖ Remove and place meringues from sheet on serving plates.
- ❖ Evenly distribute the peaches in the center of the meringues and serve.
- ❖ Place some leftover meringue in a lined jar for up to 1 week at room temperature.

119) Rhubarb Crumble

Preparation Time: 15 minutes   **Cooking Time**: 30 minutes   **Servings: 6**

Ingredients:

- ✓ 2 tablespoons water
- ✓ 2 tablespoons granulated sugar
- ✓ 2 apples, peeled, cored and thinly sliced
- ✓ 1 cup chopped rhubarb
- ✓ ½ cup unsalted butter, room temperature

Directions:

- ❖ Preheat the oven to about 325°F.
- ❖ Lightly oil a buttered 8-by-8-inch baking dish; set aside.
- ❖ Mix the rice, sugar and cinnamon in a small bowl until well blended.
- ❖ Rub the dough between your fingertips and apply the butter so that it resembles coarse crumbs.

Ingredients:

- ✓ ½ teaspoon ground cinnamon
- ✓ ½ cup of brown sugar
- ✓ 1 cup all-purpose flour
- ✓ Unsalted butter to grease the pan.

- ❖ Mix rhubarb, apple, sugar and water in a medium saucepan over medium heat and simmer for about 20 minutes or until rhubarb is tender.
- ❖ Across the baking bowl, pour in the fruit mixture and finish with the crumble evenly.
- ❖ Bake for 20-30 minutes or until crumble is golden brown. Serve hot.

120) Fresh parfait

Preparation Time: 10 minutes   **Cooking Time**: None   **Servings: 6**

Ingredients:

- ✓ Four cups of fat-free yogurt
- ✓ Stevia, 3 tablespoons.
- ✓ Two tablespoons of lime juice

Directions:

- ❖ Mix the yogurt with the stevia, lime juice, lime zest and mint in a bowl and stir.

Ingredients:

- ✓ Two teaspoons of lime zest, grind
- ✓ Four grapefruits, chopped and peeled
- ✓ Cut 1 tablespoon of spices
- ❖ Divide grapefruits into small cups, add each to yogurt mixture and serve.

121) Delicious peach pie

Preparation Time: 10 minutes   **Cooking Time**: 20 minutes   **Servings: 4**

Ingredients:

- ✓ Two peaches, peeled and sliced
- ✓ ½ cup of raspberries
- ✓ ½ teaspoon of coconut sugar
- ✓ Three eggs, beaten

Directions:

- ❖ In a bowl, comb the peaches with the sugar and raspberries.
- ❖ In another bowl, mix the eggs with the milk and flour and beat.

Ingredients:

- ✓ Avocado oil, 1 tablespoon
- ✓ ½ cup of almond milk
- ✓ ½ cup whole wheat flour
- ✓ ¼ cup of fat-free yogurt
- ❖ Grease a cake pan with oil, insert egg mixture, then peaches, scatter, bake at 400 degrees F for twenty minutes, slice and serve.

122) Simple Brownies

Preparation Time: 30 minutes   **Cooking Time**: None   **Servings**: 8

Ingredients:

- ✓ Dark chocolate Six ounces, diced
- ✓ Four egg whites
- ✓ 1/2 cup of hot water
- ✓ Extract 1 teaspoon of vanilla
- ✓ 2/3 cup sugar for the coconut

Directions:

- ❖ Integrate the chocolate and hot water into a cup and shake very well.
- ❖ Apply the vanilla extract and egg whites and mix well again.
- ❖ Integrate the sugar with the flour, baking powder and nuts in another pan. Stir.

Ingredients:

- ✓ One and 1/2 full cup of flour
- ✓ 1/2 cup sliced walnuts
- ✓ Kitchen spray
- ✓ 1 tablespoon baking powder

- ❖ Combine the two mixtures, mix well, place in a cake pan greased with cooking spray, spread well, bake for 30 minutes in the oven, cool, cut and serve.

123) Apple Tart

Preparation Time: 15 minutes   **Cooking Time**: 25 minutes   **Servings**: 8

Ingredients:

- ✓ Four apples, diced and cut into pieces
- ✓ 1/4 cup of natural apple juice
- ✓ Cranberries per 1/2 cup, dried
- ✓ Two tablespoons of cornstarch
- ✓ Two teaspoons of coconut sugar
- ✓ Extract 1 teaspoon of vanilla

Directions:

- ❖ Supplement blueberries with apple juice in a cup.
- ❖ Supplement apples with cornstarch in another pan, swirl and apply blueberry mixture.
- ❖ Mix everything together, add the vanilla and cinnamon, and then mix again.

Ingredients:

- ✓ 1/4 teaspoon dry cinnamon
  As for the crust:
- ✓ A cup and a quarter of whole wheat flour
- ✓ Two teaspoons of sugar
- ✓ Coconut oil for three teaspoons, melted
- ✓ 1/4 cup of ice water

- ❖ Sift the flour with the sugar, oil and cooled water into another bowl and mix until the dough is finished.
- ❖ Shift dough, flatten well, roll into a circle and move to a pastry pan on a workpiece surface.
- ❖ Push crust well into baking dish, pour apple mixture over crust, place in oven, bake for 25 minutes at 375 °F, and lower temperature, slice and serve.

PART II: INTRODUCTION

A diet deficient in phosphorus, protein, and sodium is a renal diet. A renal diet often emphasizes the value of eating high-quality protein and typically limiting fluids.

To decrease the amount of waste in the blood, individuals with impaired kidney function must adhere to a renal or kidney diet. Waste in the blood is produced by the liquids and foods that are ingested. Because kidney activity is impaired, the kidneys do not adequately filter or extract the waste. It will negatively affect a patient's electrolyte levels if excess remains in the blood. Maintaining a renal diet can help improve kidney function and delay the progression of kidney failure.

Substances essential for screening to support a renal diet are sodium, protein, potassium, and phosphorus.

FOODS INCLUDED IN THE RENAL DIET
- Rice, wheat, bajra, corn, supa, fusali.
- Milk, curd, buttermilk.
- Toast, idli, dosa, chapati, puri, kachori, bhakri, paratha.
- All types of legumes.
- All kinds of vegetables except tomato and brinjal.
- Sweet dishes (gulab jamun, fry bread, halwa, pakoda, curdi, rasgula, etc.).
- Sweets, kulfi, peda, etc.
- Jaggery and its candies.
- Sugar, salt, ghee.
- All kinds of condiments and spices.
- Dried fruits and nuts.
- Nuts such as cashews, coconut, peanuts.
- Ghee, oil, gelatin, turmeric.
- Meat and coconut milk.
- Any kind of fish.
- Any kind of meat.
- Tofu.
- Boiled potatoes, boiled sweet potatoes, boiled white potatoes,
- Anything that is fried.
- Any kind of vegetable made with wheat flour.
- Whole wheat, rye, oats.
- Foods that should not be eaten
- Helps control urine production

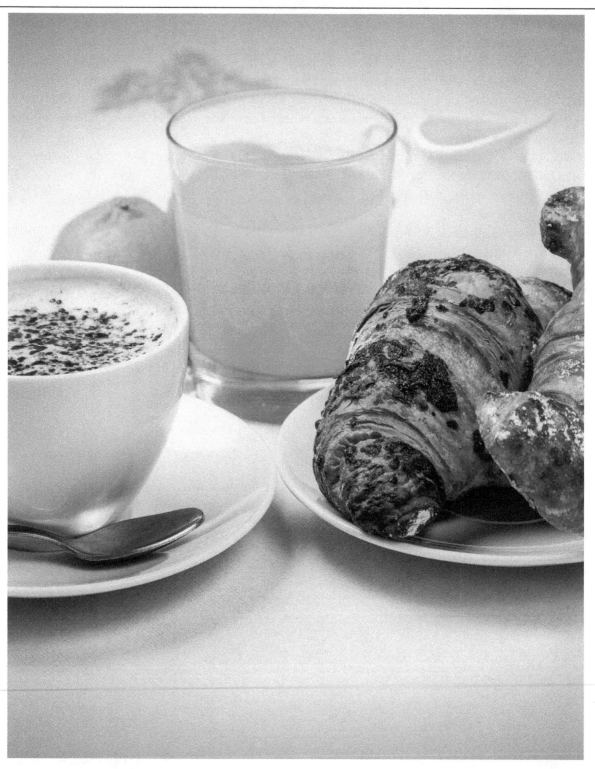

124)   Cranberry Oatmeal Cookies for Breakfast

Preparation Time:15 minutes   **Cooking Time:**20 minutes   **Servings: 12**

Ingredients:

- ✓ 1/2 cup of dried blueberries
- ✓ 3 cups rolled oats
- ✓ 1 cup of apple juice
- ✓ 1/4 teaspoon salt
- ✓ 1/2 teaspoon of cinnamon
- ✓ 1 teaspoon of vanilla extract

Directions:

- ❖ Melt the butter at room temperature. Preheat oven to about 350° F. Line baking sheet with baking paper.
- ❖ Cream the butter and sugar with a hand mixer. Add the vanilla extract, egg, protein powder, flour, salt and cinnamon to the mixture. Mix to combine.
- ❖ Stir in the applesauce. Now add the oats and cranberries and stir.

Ingredients:

- ✓ 1-1/2 ounces of vanilla whey protein powder
- ✓ 1/4 cup all-purpose flour
- ✓ 1 large egg
- ✓ 1/2 cup granulated sugar
- ✓ 1/2 cup unsalted butter

- ❖ Spread 1/4 cup of cookie dough onto the baking sheet. Lightly flatten each cookie.
- ❖ Bake until the cookies are nicely browned but still tender, about 12-15 minutes.
- ❖ Let the cookies cool on the baking sheet for about 5 minutes before moving them to the rack to cool completely.

125)   Curried egg pita pockets

Preparation Time:15 minutes   **Cooking Time:**5 minutes   **Servings: 4**

Ingredients:

- ✓ 1 cup coarsely chopped watercress
- ✓ 3 eggs, beaten
- ✓ 2 plain pita bread pockets (4 inches), halved
- ✓ ½ red bell pepper, finely chopped
- ✓ ½ teaspoon ground ginger

Directions:

- ❖ Whisk shallots, eggs, and red pepper in a large bowl until well blended.
- ❖ Melt butter in a large nonstick skillet over medium-high heat.
- ❖ Pour your egg mixture into your pan and then cook, turning the pan but not stirring, for about 3 minutes or until your eggs are just set. Remove your eggs from the heat and set aside.

Ingredients:

- ✓ 1 teaspoon of curry powder
- ✓ 2 tablespoons of light sour cream
- ✓ 2 teaspoons of unsalted butter
- ✓ ½ cup of julienned English cucumber
- ✓ 1 shallot, both the green and white parts, finely chopped
- ❖ Mix together the ginger, curry powder and sour cream in a small bowl until well blended.
- ❖ Divide the curry sauce evenly among the four halves of your pita bread, placing it on one inner side.
- ❖ Divide the watercress and cucumber similarly between the bread halves.
- ❖ To eat, place the eggs in half, separating the mixture equally.

126) Egg and vegetable muffins

Preparation Time: 15 minutes   **Cooking Time:** 20 minutes   **Servings: 4**

Ingredients:
- ✓ Pinch of freshly ground black pepper
- ✓ Pinch of red pepper flakes
- ✓ 4 eggs
- ✓ ½ red bell pepper, finely chopped

Directions:
- ❖ Preheat the oven to about 350°F.
- ❖ Spray with cooking spray on four muffin pans; set aside.
- ❖ Whisk the eggs, milk, onion, red bell pepper, parsley, red pepper flakes and black pepper together in a large bowl until well mixed.

Ingredients:
- ✓ ½ sweet onion, finely chopped
- ✓ 1 tablespoon fresh parsley chopped
- ✓ 2 tablespoons of unsweetened rice milk
- ✓ Cooking spray, for greasing muffin pans
- ❖ In the prepared muffin pans, add the egg mixture.
- ❖ Bake for 18-20 minutes or until golden brown and muffins are puffy.
- ❖ Serve cold or warm.

127) Scrambled eggs with cheese and fresh herbs

Preparation Time: 15 minutes   **Cooking Time:** 10 minutes   **Servings: 4**

Ingredients:
- ✓ Freshly ground black pepper
- ✓ 2 tablespoons unsalted butter
- ✓ 1 tablespoon fresh tarragon chopped
- ✓ 1 tablespoon finely chopped shallot, green part only

Directions:
- ❖ Beat the eggs, egg whites, cream cheese, rice milk, shallots and tarragon together in a medium bowl until well mixed and creamy.

Ingredients:
- ✓ ¼ cup unsweetened rice milk
- ✓ ½ cup cream cheese, room temperature
- ✓ 2 egg whites, at room temperature
- ✓ 3 eggs, room temperature
- ❖ Melt butter in a large skillet over medium-high heat, stirring to evenly cover the pan.
- ❖ Pour in egg mixture and cook, stirring, until eggs are thick and curds are creamy, or about 5 minutes. Add the spice seasoning and enjoy.

128) Omelette of summer vegetables

Preparation Time: 15 min   **Cooking Time**: 10 min   **Servings: 3**

Ingredients:

- ✓ Freshly ground black pepper
- ✓ ½ cup chopped and boiled red bell pepper
- ✓ Olive oil spray, for greasing the pan
- ✓ 2 tablespoons water

Ingredients:

- ✓ 2 tablespoons of chopped fresh parsley
- ✓ 1 egg
- ✓ ¼ cup chopped shallots, both the green and white parts
- ✓ 4 egg whites

Directions:

- ❖ Beat egg whites, egg, parsley and water together in a small bowl until well blended; set aside.
- ❖ Generously spray a large nonstick skillet with a splash of olive oil and set it over medium-high heat.
- ❖ Sauté shallots and peppers for about 3 minutes or until tender.

- ❖ Pour the egg mixture over the vegetables in the pan, cook for about 2 minutes, stir the pan, or start setting the edges of the egg.
- ❖ For about 4 minutes or until the omelet is set, proceed to lift and cook the egg.
- ❖ Using a spatula, loosen the omelet and fold it in half. Break off three parts of the folded omelet and pass the omelets to serving plates.
- ❖ Add black pepper for seasoning and eating.

129) French toast stuffed with strawberry cream cheese

Preparation Time: 20 min   **Cooking Time**: 1 hour and 15 min   **Servings: 4**

Ingredients:

- ✓ ¼ teaspoon ground cinnamon
- ✓ 1 tablespoon of granulated sugar
- ✓ 1 teaspoon of pure vanilla extract
- ✓ ½ cup unsweetened rice milk
- ✓ 2 eggs, beaten

Ingredients:

- ✓ 8 slices of thick white bread
- ✓ 4 tablespoons of strawberry jam
- ✓ ½ cup plain cream cheese
- ✓ Cooking spray, for greasing the pan

Directions:

- ❖ Preheat the oven to about 350°F.
- ❖ Use cooking spray to spray an 8-by-8-inch baking pan and set aside.
- ❖ Mix cream cheese and gelatin in a small bowl until well blended.
- ❖ To make sandwiches, spread 3 teaspoons of the cream cheese mixture on 4 slices of bread and top with the remaining 4 slices.
- ❖ Beat the eggs, milk and vanilla in a medium bowl until smooth.

- ❖ In the egg mixture, dip the buns and arrange them in the baking dish.
- ❖ On top of buns, pour remaining egg mixture and sprinkle with sugar and cinnamon equally.
- ❖ Cover the dish and refrigerate overnight with tape.
- ❖ Bake the wrapped French toast for 1 hour.
- ❖ Remove foil and bake until French toast is crisp, or for an additional 5 minutes.
- ❖ Serve hot.

130)   Pancakes baked in the pan

Preparation Time: 15 min   **Cooking Time**: 20 min   **Servings**: 2

Ingredients:
- ✓ Pinch of ground nutmeg
- ✓ 2 eggs
- ✓ ¼ teaspoon ground cinnamon

Directions:
- ❖ Preheat the oven to about 450°F.
- ❖ Whisk together the eggs and rice milk in a medium dish.
- ❖ Include the rice, cinnamon and nutmeg when combined, but still a little lumpy, but don't over mix.
- ❖ Use cooking spray to spray a 9-inch baking pan and place the pan for 5 minutes in the preheated oven.

Ingredients:
- ✓ ½ cup all-purpose flour
- ✓ ½ cup unsweetened rice milk
- ✓ Cooking spray, for greasing the pan
- ❖ Gently pull out the pan and place the pancake batter in the pan.
- ❖ Return the pan to the oven and bake the pancake for about 20 minutes or until the sides are puffy and crispy.
- ❖ To eat, split the pancake in half.

131)   Egg in the hole

Preparation Time: 5 min   **Cooking Time**: 5 min   **Servings**: 2

Ingredients:
- ✓ Freshly ground black pepper
- ✓ Pinch of cayenne pepper
- ✓ 2 tablespoons of chopped fresh chives

Directions:
- ❖ Cut a 2-inch round from the center of each piece of bread using a cookie cutter or small bottle.
- ❖ Melt butter in a large nonstick skillet over medium-high heat.
- ❖ In the skillet, place the bread, toast it for 1 minute and then turn the bread over. Done.

Ingredients:
- ✓ 2 eggs
- ✓ ¼ cup unsalted butter
- ✓ 2 (½ inch thick) slices of Italian bread
- ❖ In the center of the loaf, crack the eggs into the holes and bake for about 2 minutes or until the eggs are set and the bread is golden brown.
- ❖ Top with chopped chives, black pepper and cayenne pepper.
- ❖ For another 2 minutes, bake the bread.
- ❖ In each serving dish, pass an egg through the hole.

132)   Fruit and Cheese Breakfast Wrap

Preparation Time: 10 min   **Cooking Time**: None   **Servings**: 2

Ingredients:
- ✓ 1 tablespoon of honey
- ✓ 1 apple, peeled, pitted and thinly sliced

Directions:
- ❖ On a dry work surface, lay out all of the tortillas and sprinkle 1 tablespoon cream cheese over each tortilla, leaving about 1/2 inch around the edges.
- ❖ On the cream cheese, just off the center of the tortilla on the side closest to you, place the apple slices, leaving about 11/2 inches on either side and 2 inches on the edge.

Ingredients:
- ✓ 2 tablespoons plain cream cheese
- ✓ 2 flour tortillas (6 inches)

- ❖ Gently drizzle the apples with the honey.
- ❖ Fold the left and right sides of the tortillas to the center, placing the side over the apples.
- ❖ Fold it over the fruit and side pieces, choosing the edge of the tortilla closest to you. Roll up the tortilla to build a tight wrap away from you.
- ❖ With the second tortilla, repeat.

133) Pancakes baked in the pan

Preparation Time: 15 min   **Cooking Time**: 20 min   **Servings: 2**

Ingredients:
- ✓ Pinch of ground nutmeg
- ✓ 2 eggs
- ✓ ¼ teaspoon ground cinnamon

Directions:
- ❖ Preheat the oven to about 450°F.
- ❖ Whisk together the eggs and rice milk in a medium dish.
- ❖ Include the rice, cinnamon and nutmeg when combined, but still a little lumpy, but don't over mix.
- ❖ Use cooking spray to spray a 9-inch baking pan and place the pan for 5 minutes in the preheated oven.

Ingredients:
- ✓ ½ cup all-purpose flour
- ✓ ½ cup unsweetened rice milk
- ✓ Cooking spray, for greasing the pan
- ❖ Gently pull out the pan and place the pancake batter in the pan.
- ❖ Return the pan to the oven and bake the pancake for about 20 minutes or until the sides are puffy and crispy.
- ❖ To eat, split the pancake in half.

134) Egg in the hole

Preparation Time: 5 min   **Cooking Time**: 5 min   **Servings: 2**

Ingredients:
- ✓ Freshly ground black pepper
- ✓ Pinch of cayenne pepper
- ✓ 2 tablespoons of chopped fresh chives

Directions:
- ❖ Cut a 2-inch round from the center of each piece of bread using a cookie cutter or small bottle.
- ❖ Melt butter in a large nonstick skillet over medium-high heat.
- ❖ In the skillet, place the bread, toast it for 1 minute and then turn the bread over. Done.

Ingredients:
- ✓ 2 eggs
- ✓ ¼ cup unsalted butter
- ✓ 2 (½ inch thick) slices of Italian bread
- ❖ In the center of the loaf, crack the eggs into the holes and bake for about 2 minutes or until the eggs are set and the bread is golden brown.
- ❖ Top with chopped chives, black pepper and cayenne pepper.
- ❖ For another 2 minutes, bake the bread.
- ❖ In each serving dish, pass an egg through the hole.

135) Fruit and Cheese Breakfast Wrap

Preparation Time: 10 min   **Cooking Time**: None   **Servings: 2**

Ingredients:
- ✓ 1 tablespoon of honey
- ✓ 1 apple, peeled, pitted and thinly sliced

Directions:
- ❖ On a dry work surface, lay out all of the tortillas and sprinkle 1 tablespoon cream cheese over each tortilla, leaving about 1/2 inch around the edges.
- ❖ On the cream cheese, just off the center of the tortilla on the side closest to you, place the apple slices, leaving about 1 1/2 inches on either side and 2 inches on the edge.

Ingredients:
- ✓ 2 tablespoons plain cream cheese
- ✓ 2 flour tortillas (6 inches)

- ❖ Gently drizzle the apples with the honey.
- ❖ Fold the left and right sides of the tortillas to the center, placing the side over the apples.
- ❖ Fold it over the fruit and side pieces, choosing the edge of the tortilla closest to you. Roll up the tortilla to build a tight wrap away from you.
- ❖ With the second tortilla, repeat.

136) Blueberry muffins with cinnamon and nutmeg

Preparation Time: 15-20 min   **Cooking Time**: 15 min   **Servings: 4**

Ingredients:

- ✓ 2½ cups of fresh blueberries
- ✓ 2 tablespoons of pure vanilla extract
- ✓ ½ cup of canola oil
- ✓ Pinch of ground ginger
- ✓ ½ teaspoon ground nutmeg
- ✓ 1 teaspoon ground cinnamon

Directions:

- ❖ Preheat the oven to about 375°F.
- ❖ Cover ramekins with paper liners of a muffin pan; set aside.
- ❖ Mix rice milk and vinegar in a small bowl; set aside for 10 minutes.
- ❖ Mix the flour, sugar, baking soda, cinnamon, nutmeg and ginger in a large bowl until well combined. To balance the milk mixture, include the oil and vanilla and whisk to combine.
- ❖ To the dry ingredients, apply the milk mixture and beat until just blended.

Ingredients:

- ✓ 1 tablespoon baking soda substitute Enter-G
- ✓ 1 cup granulated sugar
- ✓ 3½ cups all-purpose flour
- ✓ 1 tablespoon apple cider vinegar
- ✓ 2 cups of unsweetened rice milk

- ❖ Fold blueberries into it. Spread evenly over the ramekins with the muffin batter.
- ❖ Bake the muffins for 25-30 minutes or until a toothpick inserted into the center of the muffin comes out clean, introducing the gold.
- ❖ Allow muffins to cool before serving for 15 minutes.
- ❖ Serve hot.

137) Banana-Nut Oatmeal

Preparation Time: 15 min   **Cooking Time**: None   **Servings: 4**

Ingredients:

- ✓ A cup of steel cut oats
- ✓ One banana, puree
- ✓ 1/3 of a cup of walnuts, sliced
- ✓ Two cups of skimmed milk
- ✓ Two cups of water
- ✓ 1/3 of a cup of honey

Directions:

- ❖ Add all ingredients to a slow cooker. Stir gently, cover and simmer for eight hours.

Ingredients:

- ✓ Two teaspoons of cinnamon.
- ✓ 1/2 teaspoon of nutmeg
- ✓ 1 teaspoon vanilla extract.
- ✓ 1/2 of a teaspoon of salt

- ❖ Offer over the addition of sliced bananas and walnuts.

138)   Homemade Greek yogurt

Preparation Time: 10 min   **Cooking Time**: 10 min   **Servings: 8**

Ingredients:

- ✓ 1/2 gallon of 2% milk
- ✓ One cup of condensed milk (this is voluntary but thickens the yogurt)
- ✓ 1/2 cup of live yogurt culture (can use plain plain yogurt pure)

Ingredients:

- ✓ Thermometer
- ✓ Small blanket
- ✓ For spreading cheesecloth

Directions:

- ❖ Add milk to a saucepan over low heat. Stir in milk powder. Heat milk slowly; cook until it reaches 180°F (about 1-2 hours, depending on your stove). 3. Turn off the slow stove and cool the milk to 110°F. Stir in live Culture yogurt and stir once completely melted. Wrap the slow stove (which has been turned off) to maintain heat inside a blanket. Leave there for 6-8 hours.
- ❖ Remove the lid from the slow cooker. You may need to soak to make a thick, Greek-style yogurt to create whey (the substance on top of the cream) from the yogurt.

- ❖ Put a number to make this; in a strainer, layer cheesecloth. On top of a large bowl, place the strainer. Add the yogurt to the strainer and let it drain for a few hours in the refrigerator before draining. The continuity you need has been hit. You now have a delicious Greek yogurt!
- ❖ In mason jars (or other containers) pour yogurt and place in refrigerator for 7-10 days.

139)   Breakfast casserole

Preparation Time: 10 min   **Cooking Time**: 10 min   **Servings: 8**

Ingredients:

- ✓ Frozen pancakes for 4 cups
- ✓ Twelve eggs
- ✓ 1/2 cup of low-fat milk
- ✓ Ten ounces of prepared, low-sodium sausage
- ✓ Cheddar cheese - 8 ounces, shredded

Ingredients:

- ✓ Two garlic cloves, diced
- ✓ One strong onion, chopped
- ✓ 1/2 red bell pepper, chopped
- ✓ Freshly ground black pepper

Directions:

- ❖ Spray the edge of a slow stove with cooking spray.
- ❖ Beat the eggs in a large dish. Stir in milk, and mustard, black pepper, and turn until well mixed.
- ❖ Place in bottom of slow stove with 1/2 hash browns. Top with 1/2 of each: sausage, bell bell pepper, cheese, garlic, onion.

- ❖ Place second layer of browns, sausage rolls, hash browns, bell bell pepper, cheese, garlic, and onion.
- ❖ Place beaten egg on top of layers. Cover and simmer for 4 to 5 hours. Up to 2 to 3 hours before eggs are done.

140) Almond butter and banana toast

Preparation Time: 10 min   **Cooking Time**: 7 min   **Servings**: 1

Ingredients:

- ✓ 2 slices of 100% wholemeal bread
- ✓ Macadamia nuts 2 tablespoons.

Directions:

- ❖ Toast the bread and sprinkle the macadamia nuts on each piece.

Ingredients:

- ✓ One small banana, cut
- ✓ 1/8 teaspoon ground cinnamon
- ❖ On top, place the banana slices and sprinkle with cinnamon.

141) English muffin with berries

Preparation Time: 5 min   **Cooking Time**: 5 min   **Servings**: 1

Ingredients:

- ✓ English muffin made with 100% whole wheat, cut in half
- ✓ One cup of reduced fat cream cheese

Directions:

- ❖ Toast the English muffin halves.

Ingredients:

- ✓ Four thinly sliced strawberries
- ✓ 1/2 cup crushed blueberries
- ❖ Spread cream cheese on each toasted half, equally, and top with fruit.

142) Healthy English muffin Lox

Preparation Time: 15 min   **Cooking Time**: 20 min   **Servings**: 2

Ingredients:

- ✓ A 100% whole wheat English muffin, cut in half
- ✓ 1/4 of a teaspoon of fresh dill, finely chopped
- ✓ One third of a teaspoon of pure lemon juice
- ✓ Two cups of low-fat cream cheese

Directions:

- ❖ Toast the English muffin halves. In a large dish, meanwhile, the chopped dill and lemon juice are mixed equally with the cream.
- ❖ Pour cream cheese mixture evenly on each side, around toasted muffin.
- ❖ Rinse the salmon under running water to drop the canned liquid, then spread the fish evenly over the English muffin halves.

Ingredients:

- ✓ One (four ounces) of water should be wild, no salt added, washed salmon,
- ✓ Six thin, unpeeled cucumber slices
- ✓ Six thin slices of Roma tomato
- ✓ Crushed black pepper
- ❖ If the salmon is too heavy, flatten it. First, with a fork.
- ❖ Top with cucumber slices and onion, and sprinkle with pepper to taste.

143) **Bowl protein**

Preparation Time: 12 min   **Cooking Time**: None   **Servings: 1**

Ingredients:

- ✓ 3/4 cup low-fat cottage cheese
- ✓ 1/2 huge banana, thinly sliced

Ingredients:

- ✓ One tablespoon of almond butter
- ✓ 1/4 cup lightly cooked old oats

Directions:

- ❖ In a small dish, mix all the combined ingredients, and enjoy immediately.

144) **Sandwich with sausage and eggs**

Preparation Time: 5 min   **Cooking Time**: 5 min   **Servings: 1**

Ingredients:

- ✓ 1 tablespoon shredded cheddar cheese
- ✓ 1 turkey sausage
- ✓ ¼ cup of liquid egg replacer - low in cholesterol

Directions:

- ❖ Spray a small saucepan with oil and heat it.
- ❖ Pour in and heat egg replacer, turning it almost completely as it is heated.
- ❖ Toast the muffin with the toast.

Ingredients:

- ✓ 1 English muffin
- ✓ Kitchen spray

- ❖ Patty is baked in the oven.
- ❖ Fold in the egg and place, covered with the patty, in the muffin.
- ❖ Sprinkle with cheese, top with muffin top and eat

145) **Oatmeal deluxe with berries**

Preparation Time: 5 min   **Cooking Time**: 5 min   **Servings: 2**

Ingredients:

- ✓ One 1/2 cup of unsweetened pure almond milk
- ✓ 1/8 teaspoon of vanilla extract
- ✓ 1 cup old fashioned oats

Directions:

- ❖ In a shallow saucepan, heat the almond milk and vanilla over medium heat.
- ❖ Insert the oats and stir for about four minutes, or until most of the liquid has drained, so that the solution begins to simmer.

Ingredients:

- ✓ 3/4 cup coarsely chopped blackberry, blueberry and strawberry mixture
- ✓ Two tablespoons of toasted pecans
- ❖ Stir in the berries.
- ❖ Scoop out 2 bowls of the mixture and finish with the toasted pecans.

146) Oatmeal with apples and cinnamon

Preparation Time: 5 min   **Cooking Time**: 8 min   **Servings: 2**

Ingredients:

- ✓ One 1/2 cup of unsweetened pure almond milk
- ✓ Old oats for 1 cup
- ✓ One large, unpeeled Granny Smith apple, cut into cubes

Directions:

- ❖ Place the milk over medium heat until boiling, and then include the oats and apple.
- ❖ Stir until most of the liquid is absorbed, about four minutes.

Ingredients:

- ✓ 1/4 teaspoon ground cinnamon
- ✓ Two tablespoons of toasted walnut pieces

- ❖ Stir in the cinnamon.
- ❖ Spread the oatmeal combination into two compartments and then top with the nuts.

147) Energy of Oatmeal

Preparation Time: 5 min   **Cooking Time**: 8 min   **Servings: 1**

Ingredients:

- ✓ 1/4 cup water
- ✓ 1/4 cup of low-fat milk
- ✓ Old fashioned oats, half cup
- ✓ Four white eggs, pounded

Directions:

- ❖ In a small saucepan, heat the water and milk to a boil over medium heat.
- ❖ Include oats, stirring constantly, or until most of the moisture is drained, about four minutes.
- ❖ Apply the beaten egg steadily, stirring continuously.

Ingredients:

- ✓ 1/8 teaspoon ground cinnamon
- ✓ 1/8 teaspoon ground ginger
- ✓ 1/4 cup blueberries

- ❖ Cook for the next five minutes just until the eggs are no longer runny.
- ❖ Through the oatmeal mixture, whisk in the cinnamon and ginger and sweep the mixture into a cup.
- ❖ Top with berries and serve immediately.

148) Anna's Organic Granola

Preparation Time: 5 min   **Cooking Time**: 10 min   **Servings: 12**

Ingredients:

- ✓ Three cups of old-fashioned oats
- ✓ 1/4 cup of flaxseed
- ✓ One cup of diced almonds
- ✓ 1/2 teaspoon ground cinnamon
- ✓ 1/4 teaspoon ground ginger
- ✓ 1/4 cup brown sugar

Directions:

- ❖ Preheat the oven to 250°F.
- ❖ In a spacious cup, combine the first 6 elements and stir to integrate effectively.
- ❖ Place the maple syrup or honey, oil and almond extraction in another shallow dish.
- ❖ Drop the wet ingredients into the dry ingredients and combine when there are no more dry areas, evenly with a spatula.

Ingredients:

- ✓ 1/4 cup honey or maple syrup
- ✓ 1/4 cup extra virgin olive oil
- ✓ 1/2 teaspoon of almond extract
- ✓ 1 cup golden grapes
- ✓ A mist of olive oil

- ❖ Place in 2 greased baking dishes. Bake for about 1 hour and 15 minutes, turning once every 15 minutes to get an even shade.
- ❖ While blending, divide the granola chunks to get the perfect consistency. Remove from oven and transfer to a large bowl.
- ❖ Stir in the raisins so that they are evenly dispersed.

149) Hot quinoa and berries

Preparation Time: 10 min   **Cooking Time**: 15-20 min   **Servings: 2**

Ingredients:

- ✓ One cup of uncooked quinoa
- ✓ One cup unsweetened coconut milk
- ✓ One cup of water

Directions:

- ❖ Rinse quinoa (if not pre-rinsed).
- ❖ Place the quinoa, coconut milk and water over low heat in a small covered kettle.
- ❖ Reduce the heat to low and simmer for 10-15 minutes until the liquid has been consumed.

Ingredients:

- ✓ 1/2 cup of assorted blackberries
- ✓ Two tablespoons of sliced toasted pecans
- ✓ Two tablespoons of raw sugar, additional
- ❖ Cooked quinoa should be slightly al dente; it is able to do this because most of the grains have unrolled and you will see the germ unrolled.
- ❖ Allow the quinoa to sit in the cover pot for about five minutes.
- ❖ Smear softly with a spoon and sweep into two serving containers, and top with blackberries, pecans and honey (if using).

150) Fruit milk parfait

Preparation Time: 7 min   **Cooking Time**: None   **Servings: 1**

Ingredients:

- ✓ A cup of plain low-fat Greek yogurt
- ✓ 1/4 cup blueberries
- ✓ 1/4 cup diced kiwi fruit

Directions:

- ❖ Place half of the yogurt in a shallow glass container or parfait tray.
- ❖ Top with a light layer of blueberries, flaxseed meal, kiwi, strawberries and granola.

Ingredients:

- ✓ 1/4 cup of diced strawberries
- ✓ 1 tablespoon ground flaxseed meal or flaxseed meal
- ✓ 1/2 cup (or Anna's Homemade Granola) of low-calorie granola
- ❖ Layer and top the leftover fruit, flax seeds and granola with the leftover yogurt.

151) Yogurt with banana and almonds

Preparation Time: 5 min   **Cooking Time**: 5 min   **Servings: 1**

Ingredients:

- ✓ 1 tablespoon raw, crunchy, unsalted almond butter
- ✓ 3/4 cup plain Greek low-fat yogurt
- ✓ 1/4 cup old-fashioned oats, lightly cooked

Directions:

- ❖ In the oven, melt the almond butter for 15 seconds.

Ingredients:

- ✓ 1/2 large blunt banana
- ✓ 1/8 teaspoon of cinnamon powder

- ❖ Put the yogurt in a cup and mix in the almond butter, oats and bananas.
- ❖ Sprinkle cinnamon over the top.

152) Open breakfast sandwich

Preparation Time: 5 min   **Cooking Time**: 10 min   **Servings: 1**

Ingredients:
- ✓ One 1/2 teaspoon of pure quality olive oil
- ✓ Two egg whites, crushed
- ✓ Spinach 1/2 cup
- ✓ Cracked black pepper, to suit

Directions:
- ❖ Preheat oven or toaster oven to 400°F. Heat a small nonstick skillet over medium heat.
- ❖ Apply the oil to the pan and then add the egg whites when the oil is hot.
- ❖ While frying, crumble the eggs, then introduce the spinach and sprinkle with pepper to taste.

Ingredients:
- ✓ 1 teaspoon of brown mustard
- ✓ A strip of 100% whole wheat bread
- ✓ Two large tomato cuts
- ✓ A small slice of low-fat cheddar cheese
- ❖ Spread mustard on bread and insert tomatoes and scrambled eggs, and top with cheese.
- ❖ Heat until cheese is melted, about two minutes in the oven.

153) Scramble for the Mediterranean

Preparation Time: 5 min   **Cooking Time**: 8 min   **Servings: 1**

Ingredients:
- ✓ Two tablespoons of pure olive oil extra
- ✓ 1/8 cup chopped red onion
- ✓ One garlic with a moderate clove, diced
- ✓ 1/4 cup chopped red bell pepper
- ✓ 1/4 cup canned artichoke hearts, rinsed and discarded, chopped

Directions:
- ❖ Over medium heat, heat a mini nonstick skillet.
- ❖ Apply oil to hot skillet and introduce onion and garlic while oil is hot. Cook for 1 minute before inserting the bell bell pepper strips and artichoke hearts. Sauté the vegetables for three more minutes, just until the bell bell pepper is smooth and the onion is translucent.

Ingredients:
- ✓ Two white eggs
- ✓ One whole egg
- ✓ 1/8 teaspoon. dried oregano
- ✓ 1/8 crushed black pepper Teaspoon.
- ✓ 1/8 cup low-fat feta cheese

- ❖ In a small skillet, mix the egg whites and eggs in a bowl and season with the oregano and black pepper.
- ❖ Add the eggs and mix with a Spatula combination. Run for 3 to 4 minutes or until eggs are no longer runny.
- ❖ Remove from heat, top with feta and cover until feta is set.
- ❖ melt. Serve immediately.

154) Vegetarian omelette

Preparation Time: 5 min   **Cooking Time**: 10 min   **Servings: 1**

Ingredients:

- ✓ One tablespoon of pure extra olive oil
- ✓ 1/4 cup of coarsely sliced broccoli
- ✓ Two tablespoons of chopped red onion
- ✓ One clove of chopped garlic
- ✓ Sawn 1/4 cup zucchini

Directions:

- ❖ On low pressure, heat a medium-sized bowl without a stick, and add the oil as the pan heats up.
- ❖ Insert the broccoli when the oil is hot.
- ❖ before introducing the onion, garlic and zucchini. Sauté for 3 to 4 minutes. Mix in a small cup, egg whites and whole eggs combined and season with salt or chili.

Ingredients:

- ✓ Two egg whites
- ✓ One whole egg
- ✓ 1/8 cup sliced low-fat cheddar cheese
- ✓ 1/8 teaspoon sea salt
- ✓ 1/8 crushed black pepper Teaspoon.
- ❖ Switch the heat to low and add the eggs to the container of vegetables to make sure the container is angled so that the eggs wrap around the vegetables evenly.
- ❖ Turn off the heat after 30 seconds, rotate the omelet and spread half of the omelet with the cheese.
- ❖ Fold the other half over the cheese and protect the pan with a lid. Allow to steam, or until cheese is malted, for 1 to 2 minutes.
- ❖ Serve instantly.

155) Rhubarb bread pudding

Preparation Time: 15 minutes, plus 30 minutes soaking time   **Cooking Time**: 50 min   **Servings: 6**

Ingredients:

- ✓ 2 cups chopped fresh rhubarb
- ✓ 1 vanilla pod, separated
- ✓ 3 eggs
- ✓ 1 tablespoon of cornstarch

Directions:

- ❖ Preheat the oven to about 350°F.
- ❖ Lightly oil a buttered 8-by-8-inch baking dish; set aside.
- ❖ Whisk the rice milk, eggs, sugar and cornstarch in a large dish.
- ❖ In the milk mixture, scrape in the vanilla seeds and whisk to combine.
- ❖ Apply the egg mixture to the bread and beat to completely cover the bread.

Ingredients:

- ✓ ½ cup granulated sugar
- ✓ 10 thick pieces of white bread, cut into 1 inch pieces
- ✓ 1½ cups unsweetened rice milk
- ✓ Unsalted butter to grease the pan.
- ❖ To mix, apply sliced rhubarb and stir.
- ❖ Allow the bread and egg mixture to soak for 30 minutes.
- ❖ In the prepared baking dish, pour the mixture, cover with aluminum foil and bake for 40 minutes.
- ❖ Uncover and bake bread pudding for an additional 10 minutes or until pudding is brown and set.
- ❖ Serve hot.

156) Homemade Granola

Preparation Time: 10 min **Cooking Time**: 30-40 min **Servings: 10**

Ingredients:

- ✓ 300g (10½oz) rolled oats
- ✓ 2 tablespoons of soft brown sugar
- ✓ 1 tablespoon of lemon juice

Directions:

- ❖ Preheat the oven to about 140°C (120°C fan)/275°F/gas 1.
- ❖ Gasoline, honey/syrup, lemon juice and sugar are dissolved in a large saucepan over medium heat. The goal is to not boil the mixture, but just allow the ingredients to melt and blend together. Then the oats are applied and thoroughly whisked.

Ingredients:

- ✓ 2 tablespoons of clear honey or golden syrup
- ✓ 4 tablespoons sunflower or vegetable oil
- ✓ Dried cranberries (optional)
- ❖ Spread the mixture in an even layer on a baking sheet (depending on their height, you'll need two baking sheets. Bake until crispy, about 30-40 minutes. Check the granola every 10 minutes and turn to ensure even baking.
- ❖ You could add a few handfuls of dried cranberries until they are cooked and cooled. The granola can be placed in an airtight jar and used within a month.

157) Festive berry parfait

Preparation Time: 20 minutes plus 1 hour for refrigeration **Cooking Time**: None **Servings: 4**

Ingredients:

- ✓ 1 cup fresh sliced strawberries
- ✓ 2 cups of fresh blueberries
- ✓ 1 cup crumbled meringue cookies
- ✓ ½ teaspoon ground cinnamon

Directions:

- ❖ Beat milk, sugar, cream cheese and cinnamon together in a small bowl until creamy.
- ❖ Spoon ¼ cup of the crumbled cookie into 4 glasses (6 ounces) at the bottom of each.
- ❖ On top of cakes, spoon ¼ cup of the cream cheese mixture.

Ingredients:

- ✓ 1 tablespoon of granulated sugar
- ✓ ½ cup plain cream cheese, room temperature
- ✓ 1 cup vanilla rice milk, room temperature

- ❖ Place ¼ cup berries on top of cream cheese.
- ❖ Repeat with the cookies, cream cheese and berries in each cup.
- ❖ For 1 hour, chill in refrigerator and serve.

158) Baked egg cups

Preparation Time: 10 min **Cooking Time**: 25 min **Servings: 12**

Ingredients:

- ✓ 12 eggs
- ✓ ¼ teaspoon of black pepper
- ✓ 1/3 cup mushrooms

Directions:

- ❖ Preheat oven to about 350°F and use paper liners to fill a muffin tray.
- ❖ Dice all the vegetables and cook the bacon and crumble it into the vegetables.
- ❖ Put your mixture in the cups.

Ingredients:

- ✓ 1/3 cup of bell bell pepper
- ✓ 1/3 cup onion
- ✓ 6 slices of bacon, low-sodium
- ❖ Whisk and add the eggs and pepper to the cups, leaving a little room in each.
- ❖ Bake the muffins for about 25 minutes or until they grow and firm up.
- ❖ Serve hot.

159) Healthy porridge

Preparation Time: 4-5 min   **Cooking Time**: 1-2 min   **Servings: 4**

Ingredients:
- ✓ Cinnamon sprinkling
- ✓ ½ grated apple
- ✓ 100ml water

Directions:
- ❖ In a saucepan, combine all ingredients, heat the pan and boil for about 3-4 minutes.

Ingredients:
- ✓ 100ml of skimmed milk
- ✓ 35g (1¼oz) porridge oats

- ❖ Alternatively, cook for about 1-2 minutes in the microwave, stirring at 30 second intervals.

160) Watermelon and Raspberry Smoothie

Preparation Time: 10 min   **Cooking Time**: None   **Servings: 2**

Ingredients:
- ✓ 1 cup of ice
- ✓ ½ cup fresh raspberries

Directions:
- ❖ In a blender, place cabbage and pump for 2 minutes or until finely chopped.
- ❖ Add the watermelon and raspberries and pulse until well blended, or about 1 minute.

Ingredients:
- ✓ 1 cup of diced watermelon
- ✓ ½ cup boiled, cooled and shredded red cabbage

- ❖ Until the smoothie is very rich and smooth, apply ice and blend.
- ❖ Pour in 2 glasses and serve.

161) Apple Pancake Rings

Preparation Time: 5 min   **Cooking Time**: 1-2 min   **Servings: 20**

Ingredients:
- ✓ ½ teaspoon of cinnamon
- ✓ ¾ cup of frying oil
- ✓ 1 tablespoon of canola oil
- ✓ 1/3 cup of almond milk
- ✓ 1/3 cup low fat milk 1%

Directions:
- ❖ Peel and core the apples. From each apple, cut 5 circles, 1/2" thick.
- ❖ Sift together the rice, baking powder and two teaspoons of sugar.
- ❖ In a separate dish, combine the egg, almond yogurt, milk and 1 tablespoon oil.
- ❖ Combine the egg and dry mixtures before they are combined.
- ❖ In a deep skillet, boil 1 inch of cooking oil.

Ingredients:
- ✓ 1 beaten egg
- ✓ 1 teaspoon baking powder
- ✓ 6 tablespoons of sugar
- ✓ 1 cup white flour
- ✓ 4 large cooking apples
- ❖ Dip the apple rings in the batter and fry until golden brown or 1 to 1/2 minute.
- ❖ Drain them on cloth towels.
- ❖ Combine remaining sugar with cinnamon and sprinkle over patties.

162) Apple Oatmeal with Cinnamon

Preparation Time: 7 min   **Cooking Time**: 10 min   **Servings: 8**

Ingredients:

- ✓ 2 cups steel cut oats
- ✓ Water Eight cups
- ✓ Cinnamon - 1 teaspoon.
- ✓ 1/2 teaspoon of allspice
- ✓ Nutmeg 1/2 teaspoon.

Directions:

- ❖ Spray non-stick spray on a slow stove.
- ❖ Place all the items in the pot over low heat except for the nuts. Stir enough to make a paste.

Ingredients:

- ✓ 1/4 cup brown sugar
- ✓ 1 teaspoon of vanilla extraction
- ✓ Two apples, sliced
- ✓ 1 cup of raisins
- ✓ 1/2 cup unsalted, fried, diced walnuts
- ❖ Set the pot to low and cook for eight hours.
- ❖ Offer with diced walnuts.

163) Hot mixed cereals

Preparation Time: 10 min   **Cooking Time**: 25 min   **Servings: 4**

Ingredients:

- ✓ ½ teaspoon ground cinnamon
- ✓ 6 tablespoons of plain uncooked couscous
- ✓ 1 cup peeled and sliced apple
- ✓ 2 tablespoons whole uncooked buckwheat

Directions:

- ❖ Heat the water and milk in a medium saucepan over medium-high heat.
- ❖ Bring the bulgur, buckwheat and apple to a boil.
- ❖ Lower the heat and simmer, stirring regularly, for 20-25 minutes or until the bulgur is soft.

Ingredients:

- ✓ 6 tablespoons of uncooked bulgur
- ✓ 1¼ cup of vanilla rice milk
- ✓ 2¼ cups of water

- ❖ Stir in the couscous and cinnamon and remove the casserole from the sun.
- ❖ For 10 minutes, let the pot sit, sealed, and then fluff the cereal with a fork before eating

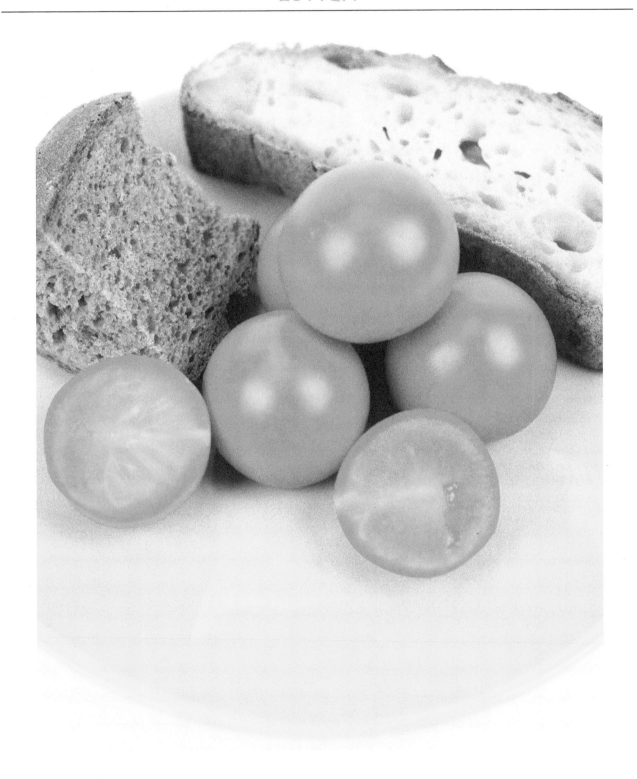

164)   Menthol lamb chops

Preparation Time: 15 min   **Cooking Time**: 15 min   **Servings: 2**

Ingredients:

- ✓ 1 tablespoon vegetable or olive oil
- ✓ 1 free-range egg, beaten
- ✓ 100g (3½oz) flour
- ✓ 2 lamb chops

Directions:

- ❖ Use a mixer to include the breadcrumbs, mint and parsley until well mixed to cook the lamb chops. Place them in a container.
- ❖ Cover the lamb chops in the starch, and then dip them until well covered in the egg and breadcrumbs. And add the spice seasoning.

Ingredients:

- ✓ 1 tablespoon fresh parsley
- ✓ 2 tablespoons fresh mint
- ✓ 100g (3½oz) breadcrumbs (homemade or brought from the store)
- ❖ Heat a medium-hot skillet. Place the lamb chops in the skillet and apply the fat. Cook for three minutes.
- ❖ Switch chops and simmer for another three minutes.
- ❖ Remove the chops and let them rest, then serve for three minutes.

165)   Chicken and lemon casserole

Preparation Time: 15-20 min   **Cooking Time**: 1 hour   **Servings: 4**

Ingredients:

- ✓ 500ml hot chicken stock with low salt content
- ✓ 2 spoons of honey
- ✓ 4 crushed garlic cloves
- ✓ 1 tablespoon vegetable or olive oil
- ✓ 80g (3oz) butter

Directions:

- ❖ Preheat the oven to about 200 degrees F (180 degrees Fan)/400 degrees F/Gas 6.
- ❖ In a bowl, place the sugar, lemon zest and lemon juice and whisk until well blended. Add the chicken pieces and stir until they are completely covered in the mixture. Set aside to marinate for at least 10 minutes.
- ❖ Heat 40g/1½ oz. butter and half the olive oil in a fireproof saucepan over medium heat. Add half of the marinated chicken parts and fry for 5-6 minutes while the butter is foaming, turning regularly, until golden brown. With the remaining butter oil and chicken parts, set the chicken parts aside, repeat and then set the chicken aside.

Ingredients:

- ✓ salt and freshly ground black pepper
- ✓ 2kg (4lb 4oz) skinless chicken thighs or drumsticks
- ✓ 1 lemon, just the zest and juice, plus a lemon cut into thin slices
- ✓ 2 teaspoons of dried thyme (optional)
- ❖ Add the garlic cloves, lemon slices, and juice from the remaining marinade to the pan and stir well, wiping any burnt pieces from the bottom of the pan with a wooden spoon. Return the cooked chicken pieces to the pan, then add the thyme and hot chicken stock and mix well. Bring the mixture to a boil and roast in the oven for 30-35 minutes, or until the chicken is cooked through and tender.
- ❖ Remove the chicken pieces from the pan and set them aside on a warm plate. Strain the sauce through a fine sieve into a saucepan, using the back of a wooden spoon to press the garlic pulp through the sieve. Simmer the lemon sauce for another 5-10 minutes over high heat or until the liquid is reduced to a thin syrup consistency.
- ❖ Spoon over chicken casserole with lemon sauce and eat.

166) Farfalle Confetti Salad

Preparation Time: 30 min plus 1 hour for refrigeration

Cooking Time: None

Servings: 6

Ingredients:

- ✓ Freshly ground black pepper.
- ✓ ½ teaspoon of granulated sugar
- ✓ 1 teaspoon fresh parsley chopped
- ✓ 1 tablespoon freshly squeezed lemon juice
- ✓ ½ cup of homemade mayonnaise
- ✓ ½ shallot, only the green part, finely chopped

Ingredients:

- ✓ 2 tablespoons of yellow bell pepper
- ✓ ¼ cup grated carrot
- ✓ ¼ cup finely chopped cucumber
- ✓ ¼ cup boiled and finely chopped red bell pepper
- ✓ 2 cups of cooked farfalle pasta

Directions:

- ❖ Combine the pasta, cucumber, red bell pepper, yellow bell pepper, carrot and shallot in a large pot.
- ❖ Whisk together the lemon juice, mayonnaise, parsley and sugar in a shallow saucepan.

- ❖ For the pasta mixture, apply the seasoning and whisk to mix. And spice the seasoning.
- ❖ Before serving, chill the salad in the refrigerator for at least 1 hour.

167) Couscous salad with spicy citrus dressing

Preparation Time: 25 min plus 1 hour for refrigeration

Cooking Time: None

Servings: 6

Ingredients:

FOR SEASONING

- ✓ Freshly ground black pepper.
- ✓ Pinch of cayenne pepper
- ✓ Zest of 1 lime
- ✓ Juice of 1 lime
- ✓ 1 tablespoon fresh parsley chopped
- ✓ 3 tablespoons freshly squeezed grapefruit juice
- ✓ ¼ cup olive oil

Ingredients:

FOR SALAD

- ✓ 1 apple, pitted and chopped
- ✓ 1 shallot, both the white and green parts, chopped
- ✓ ½ red bell pepper, chopped
- ✓ 3 cups of cooked, cooled couscous

Directions:

- ❖ TO MAKE SEASONING
- ❖ Mix grapefruit juice, olive oil, lime zest, lime juice, parsley and cayenne pepper in a shallow dish.
- ❖ Add black pepper for seasoning.

- ❖ TO MAKE SALAD
- ❖ Whisk together the red bell pepper, cooled couscous, shallots and apple in a large dish.
- ❖ For couscous mixture, apply seasoning and stir.
- ❖ Before serving, chill the salad in the refrigerator for at least 1 hour.

168)   Shepherd's pie

Preparation Time: 10 min   **Cooking Time**: 40-45 min   **Servings: 4**

Ingredients:

- ✓   ½ cup of beef sauce
- ✓   1 cup milk, 1%
- ✓   2 tablespoons of Worcestershire sauce
- ✓   ½ teaspoon of black pepper
- ✓   2 potatoes
- ✓   1 1/2 pounds of ground beef

Directions:

- ❖   Dice the onion and carrot and chop the garlic as well.
- ❖   Peel and cut potatoes into 1⁄2" cubes.
- ❖   For about 5 minutes, boil potatoes, rinse and repeat until potatoes are soft.
- ❖   In a skillet, melt half the butter and sauté the garlic and onion for about 10 minutes.
- ❖   Stir in beef and sauté until orange.
- ❖   Add the sauce, pepper, onions and Worcestershire tomato sauce.

Ingredients:

- ✓   4 tablespoons of butter
- ✓   1/3 cup of tomato sauce
- ✓   3 garlic cloves
- ✓   ¾ cup frozen peas
- ✓   1 onion
- ✓   ¾ cup of carrot
- ❖   For about 10 minutes, cook uncovered
- ❖   Preheat oven to 400 degrees F.
- ❖   With the rest of the butter, scramble the potatoes and incorporate the milk. Season with black pepper
- ❖   Spread the beef and top with the potato in a baking dish.
- ❖   Bake for about 30 minutes, until bubbles form.
- ❖   Serve with a little sauce.

169)   Apple pork chops with stuffing

Preparation Time: 10 min   **Cooking Time**: 45 min   **Servings: 6**

Ingredients:

- ✓   6 pork chops, boned
- ✓   20 ounces of apple pie filling

Directions:

- ❖   Preheat the oven to approximately 350° F.
- ❖   Spray oil on a 9" by 13" baking sheet.
- ❖   Through applying water and margarine to mixture and mixing thoroughly, make filling; set aside.

Ingredients:

- ✓   2 tablespoons of unsalted margarine
- ✓   6 ounces of low-sodium filling mixture
- ❖   Pour the pie filling over the base of the pan and place the pork chops on top of the pan.
- ❖   Cover with aluminum foil and bake for about 30 minutes.
- ❖   Remove foil; bake for the next 10 minutes and serve once heated through.

170)   Chicken or Vegetarian Curry

Preparation Time: 5-10 min   **Cooking Time**: 15-20 min   **Servings: 4**

Ingredients:
- ✓   150 ml of cream
- ✓   1 tablespoon of soft dark brown sugar
- ✓   2 tablespoons of mango chutney
- ✓   300 ml of chicken or vegetable broth
- ✓   ½ teaspoon of ginger powder
- ✓   1 medium onion
- ✓   2 tablespoons of cooking oil
- ✓   450g of chicken in 2,5 cm cubes OR 400g of chickpeas tin

Ingredients:

Seasoning
- ✓   1 teaspoon of ground cumin
- ✓   1 teaspoon of ground coriander
- ✓   1 tablespoon of spicy curry powder (use mild if you prefer)
- ✓   1 tablespoon of turmeric
- ✓   1 teaspoon of chili powder
- ✓   1 teaspoon cayenne pepper (less if you don't like spicy curry or omit it completely)
- ✓   1 teaspoon of paprika
- ✓   55g of normal flour (useless to do with chickpeas for example, 25g)

Directions:
- ❖   Mix the spice ingredients in a bowl and then add to cover the chicken or chickpeas.
- ❖   In a large heavy saucepan, heat oil, add chicken or chickpeas and cook until sealed.
- ❖   Add the ginger and onion and simmer for another 1-2 minutes.

- ❖   Stir in the broth, sugar, and chutney and bring to a boil. Cover and cook for 15 minutes, then set aside.
- ❖   Add the milk and cook, making sure the sauce does not simmer.
- ❖   Serve with boiled rice and some vegetables, preferably brown rice.

171)   Chicken and olive casserole

Preparation Time: 150 min   **Cooking Time**: 1 hour   **Servings: 4**

Ingredients:
- ✓   Pepper
- ✓   2 tablespoons of balsamic vinegar
- ✓   800g (1lb 8oz) chicken breast
- ✓   ½ teaspoon of sugar
- ✓   2 garlic cloves, minced
- ✓   1 teaspoon of dried sage
- ✓   375 ml low-salt chicken broth

Ingredients:
- ✓   ½ teaspoon of dried thyme
- ✓   400g jar of chopped tomatoes
- ✓   1 large onion, sliced
- ✓   1 cup of pickled olives (black or green or a mixture)
- ✓   1 tablespoon vegetable or olive oil

Directions:
- ❖   Steam a deep skillet, drizzle with brown chicken and oil. Set aside and remove chicken from pan.
- ❖   Cover the skillet with the onions and garlic and sauté until soft. Add the onions, chicken broth, sage, thyme, sugar, olives and balsamic vinegar. Bring to a boil and cook for a few minutes.

- ❖   Before returning the chicken to the pot, check the seasoning. For 1 hour, cover and simmer gently.
- ❖   Because it makes the chicken rough, you don't want the casserole to bubble. Just a slight bubble will give you a nice, tender poultry.
- ❖   Serve with rice and boiled vegetables.

172) Asian pear salad

Preparation Time: 30 min plus 1 hour for refrigeration   **Cooking Time**: None   **Servings: 6**

Ingredients:

- ✓ 1 teaspoon of granulated sugar
- ✓ Zest of 1 lime
- ✓ ¼ cup olive oil
- ✓ ½ red bell pepper, boiled and chopped
- ✓ 1 Asian pear, cored and grated
- ✓ 2 stalks of celery, chopped

Ingredients:

- ✓ ½ cup chopped cilantro
- ✓ 2 shallots, both green and white, chopped
- ✓ Juice of 1 lime
- ✓ 1 cup finely shredded red cabbage
- ✓ 2 cups of finely chopped green cabbage

Directions:

- ❖ Combine the red and green cabbage, celery, shallots, red bell bell pepper, pear and cilantro in a large dish.
- ❖ Mix lime juice, olive oil, lime zest and sugar in a small saucepan.

- ❖ Add the cabbage mixture to the dressing and stir to mix well.
- ❖ Before eating, chill the salad in the refrigerator for about 1 hour.

173) Frosted Cornish Hen

Preparation Time: 20 minutes   **Cooking Time**: 30 minutes   **Servings:**

Ingredients:

- ✓ 1 teaspoon of Worcestershire sauce
- ✓ 1 teaspoon Dijon mustard
- ✓ 2 tablespoons of apricot jam

Ingredients:

- ✓ 1-1/4 lb. Cornish Hen
- ✓ 3 tablespoons of butter

Directions:

- ❖ Preheat the oven to about 375° F. Melt the butter in a shallow saucepan.
- ❖ Drop and discard giblets from the cavity of a hen. Clean, rinse and dry. With a tablespoon of melted butter, massage the skin and cavity lining. Place the hen and roast in the oven for about 20 minutes.
- ❖ To remaining melted butter, stir in mustard, jam and Worcestershire sauce; heat and stir until well combined.

- ❖ Brush the hen with the apricot glaze after baking for about 20 minutes. Bake for 20-30 minutes more, and then bake every 10 minutes with the glaze. When the internal temperature exceeds 165° F, take it out of the oven.
- ❖ For 10 minutes, let hen cool, cut in half and place on serving platter. Heat leftover glaze to a boil and, before eating, pour over each serving.

174) Easy chicken and pasta

Preparation Time: 10 min   **Cooking Time**: 15 min   **Servings: 2**

Ingredients:

- ✓ 3 tablespoons of low-sodium Italian dressing
- ✓ 2 cups of cooked pasta, any shape
- ✓ 5 ounces of cooked chicken breast

Ingredients:

- ✓ 1 small zucchini olive oil
- ✓ 1/2 medium red bell pepper

Directions:

- ❖ Cut up the zucchini and bell bell pepper.
- ❖ Heat the olive oil in a non-stick skillet and sauté your bell bell pepper and zucchini until tender and crispy. Transfer to a platter.
- ❖ Cut the chicken into thin strips.

- ❖ In another skillet, heat the cooked pasta and chicken strips in the oven.
- ❖ Season the noodles with Italian seasoning. Add chicken strips and sauteed vegetables on top.

175) Veronique Chicken

Preparation Time: 10 min · · · · · · **Cooking Time**: 10 min · · · · · · **Servings: 1**

Ingredients:

- ✓ 1/4 cup heavy cream
- ✓ 1 teaspoon of dried tarragon
- ✓ 1/2 cup of green grapes without seeds
- ✓ 2 tablespoons low-sodium chicken broth
- ✓ 2 tablespoons of dry white wine

Directions:

- ❖ Heat butter in an 8-inch skillet and cook chicken breasts on all sides until golden brown. Turn out onto a platter.
- ❖ Finely chop shallots and sauté in a skillet until soft.
- ❖ Mix the cornstarch with the wine and broth in a small cup. Pour the liquid into the skillet, stir well, and then add the chicken breasts. For 5 to 6 minutes, cover and cook.

Ingredients:

- ✓ 1 teaspoon of cornstarch
- ✓ 1/2 shallot
- ✓ 2 boneless, skinless chicken breasts (4 ounces each)
- ✓ 2 tablespoons of butter
- ❖ Break the grapes in half while the chicken is simmering.
- ❖ Remove the chicken from the pan to keep warm. Keep it covered in the skillet, stir in the tarragon and cream, and heat over low heat. Stir the grapes into the sauce and simmer until fully cooked.
- ❖ Place each chicken breast on a tray. Cover with grapes and sauce.

176) Easy pork chops

Preparation Time: 15 min · · · · · · **Cooking Time**: 15 min · · · · · · **Servings: 1**

Ingredients:

- ✓ 1/4 cup of barbecue sauce
- ✓ 1-1/2 cups apple cider vinegar
- ✓ 3 cups of water

Directions:

- ❖ Preheat oven to about 300° F. Sprinkle ribs (top and bottom) evenly with seasoning.
- ❖ Use cooking spray to cover top of cooking pan; place ribs on cooking pan.
- ❖ Cover the bottom of the grill pan with water and vinegar. Place the pan with the ribs on top.

Ingredients:

- ✓ 1-1/2 lb. of baby back ribs
- ✓ 1 tablespoon of garlic-herb seasoning mix

- ❖ Place aluminum foil firmly over the ribs, tucking in along the corners. (Two pieces of foil may need to be covered properly.) This encourages the ribs to steam.
- ❖ Bake 3-1/2 to 4 hours - do not peek. Keeps steam out.
- ❖ Wipe off the foil and barbecue sauce with a brush. Cook for an additional 10 minutes in the microwave.

177) Ground beef and vegetable package in foil

Preparation Time: 10 min · · · · · · **Cooking Time**: 35 to 40 min · · · · · · **Servings: 1**

Ingredients:

- ✓ 1/4 teaspoon of black pepper
- ✓ 1/4 teaspoon of dry Italian seasoning
- ✓ 3/4 cup frozen carrots and peas

Directions:

- ❖ Preheat oven to about 375° F. Using a nonstick cooking spray, spray a sheet of aluminum foil.
- ❖ Put on the aluminum foil and mix the onion, ground beef and Worcestershire sauce into a mush.
- ❖ Add some canned peas and carrots to Patty.

Ingredients:

- ✓ 1 tablespoon Worcestershire sauce
- ✓ 4 ounces of ground beef
- ✓ 1/4 cup onion, chopped
- ❖ Sprinkle the top of the patty with a little Italian seasoning mix and black pepper.
- ❖ Sheet is folded and sealed and placed on a baking sheet. For 35 minutes, roast.
- ❖ Carefully open one end of the foil to allow steam to escape before serving.

178) Grilled cod with cucumber sauce

Preparation Time: 10 min   **Cooking Time**: 10 min   **Servings: 2**

Ingredients:

- ✓ 1 teaspoon of fresh dill
- ✓ 2 tablespoons of Greek yogurt
- ✓ 2 tablespoons of low-fat mayonnaise
- ✓ 1 lemon

Directions:

- ❖ Preheat the grill and baking pan first. Rinse the fish fillets and pat dry. Let the butter melt. Peel and thinly chop the cucumber. Cut the lemon in half and then a piece in half again. Squeeze the rest of the half.
- ❖ Mix yogurt, mayonnaise, 1 teaspoon lemon juice, chopped dill and cucumber in a shallow pan. Refrigerate until ready to consume.

Ingredients:

- ✓ 1/4 medium cucumber
- ✓ 2 tablespoons of butter
- ✓ 6 ounces of cod (2 fillets)

- ❖ Take the baking pan and cover it with cooking spray. Brush the melted butter over the fillets and sprinkle with lemon juice. For 5 minutes, cook on low heat. Drizzle with lemon juice and remaining butter and finish grilling until cooked through. Place and rotate a fork through the thickest section of the tenderloin to look for crispness. When cooked through, the meat may split quickly.
- ❖ Place each fillet with 3 tablespoons cucumber sauce on a platter. Garnish with a sprig of dill and a lemon slice.

179) Tuna noodle casserole

Preparation Time: 15 min   **Cooking Time**: 25 to 30 min   **Servings: 2**

Ingredients:

- ✓ 1/4 cup unseasoned breadcrumbs
- ✓ 1 tablespoon unsalted butter
- ✓ 1/2 cup frozen green peas
- ✓ 1/2 cup fresh sliced mushrooms

Directions:

- ❖ Preheat oven to about 350° F. According to box directions, boil egg noodles, removing salt. Drain the tuna and flake it.
- ❖ Mix the sour cream, tuna, mushrooms, cottage cheese and peas in a medium bowl.

Ingredients:

- ✓ 1/4 cup of cottage cheese
- ✓ 1/2 cup of sour cream
- ✓ 5 ounces of canned tuna in water
- ✓ 2 ounces wide egg noodles, uncooked

- ❖ Drain and stir the fried noodles into the tuna mix. Pour nonstick spray into a shallow casserole dish.
- ❖ Melt the butter in a separate bowl, then whisk in some of the breadcrumbs. Cover the casserole dish with the breadcrumbs.
- ❖ Bake until bread crumbs tend to brown, 25-30 minutes. Divide and eat in 2 servings.

180) Quick Spring Pasta

Preparation Time: 10 min   **Cooking Time**: 15-20 min   **Servings: 1**

Ingredients:
- ✓ 2 lemon wedges
- ✓ 1/2 cup of frozen whole onions
- ✓ 1 tablespoon fresh parsley
- ✓ 2 tablespoons unseasoned rice vinegar
- ✓ 1/4 cup of red bell pepper

Directions:
- ❖ Cut up the bell bell pepper and parsley.
- ❖ According to box directions, cook frozen vegetables.

Ingredients:
- ✓ 2 tablespoons of olive oil
- ✓ 1 cup of cooked tricolor spiral pasta
- ✓ 1/2 teaspoon of original herb seasoning
- ✓ 1/2 cup frozen broccoli, cauliflower and carrot mix
- ❖ Mix the vinegar, oil and herb seasoning together. Stir in cooked pasta and vegetables.
- ❖ Sprinkle with chopped parsley. With a lemon wedge, serve.

181) Waldorf Salad

Preparation Time: 20 min   **Cooking Time**: None   **Servings: 4**

Ingredients:
- ✓ 1 tablespoon of granulated sugar
- ✓ 2 tablespoons of freshly squeezed lemon juice
- ✓ ½ cup light sour cream
- ✓ 1 large apple, cored, peeled and chopped

Directions:
- ❖ On four plates, arrange lettuce evenly; set aside.
- ❖ Mix the grapes, celery and apple in a shallow dish.
- ❖ Mix the lemon juice, sour cream and sugar in another small cup.

Ingredients:
- ✓ 3 celery stalks, chopped
- ✓ 1 cup of grapes cut in half
- ✓ 3 cups of green leaf lettuce, cut into pieces

- ❖ To the grape mixture, apply the sour cream mixture and swirl to coat.
- ❖ Pour the seasoned grape mixture onto each plate, separating the mixture evenly.

182) Chili with meat

Preparation Time: 15-20 min   **Cooking Time**: 4 hours   **Servings: 8**

Ingredients:
- ✓ 1 ½ cups of water
- ✓ 2 tablespoons of chili powder
- ✓ 1 tablespoon of canola oil
- ✓ 16 ounces of stewed tomato, low sodium

Directions:
- ❖ Chop the onion, celery and peppers.
- ❖ Heat oil and fry vegetables until soft, but do not brown.
- ❖ Include beef and simmer until browned, stirring to divide.

Ingredients:
- ✓ 1 1/2 pounds of ground beef
- ✓ ½ cup green bell pepper
- ✓ 1 celery stalk
- ✓ ½ cup of onion
- ❖ Blend the tomatoes and stir them into the skillet.
- ❖ Add the water and chili powder, stir well and simmer for several hours over very low heat.

183) Chicken wrapped in bacon (or bacon) stuffed with herb cream cheese

Preparation Time: 10-15 min   **Cooking Time**: 30-35 min   **Servings: 4**

Ingredients:

- ✓ ½ teaspoon basil/organic/rosemary/thyme
- ✓ 2 tablespoons of olive oil
- ✓ 20 thin slices of bacon or your favorite bacon

Directions:

- ❖ Preheat the oven to about 200°C/400°F/Gas 6.
- ❖ Combine soft cheese with oregano, basil, rosemary and thyme in a shallow dish.
- ❖ For your chicken, make a cavity along the bottom of each chicken breast with a thin, sharp knife to create a pocket. With freshly ground black pepper, spice the chicken inside and out, then force the soft cheese mixture into the pockets.

Ingredients:

- ✓ 4 tablespoons of soft cream cheese
- ✓ 4 large skinless chicken breasts
- ✓ Blueberry sauce optional
- ❖ To flatten the stuffing slightly and close the sides, gently push each chicken breast in, then top each breast with five slices of bacon to cover completely.
- ❖ Heat the olive oil over medium heat in a large, heavy skillet, then add the chicken and cook on each side for about 2-3 minutes or until the bacon is crispy and beautifully brown. Transfer to a baking sheet and bake for about 20-25 minutes in the oven, or until the chicken is fully cooked (liquids should be clear with no sign of pink).

184) Lettuce and asparagus salad with raspberries

Preparation Time: 25 min   **Cooking Time**: None   **Servings: 4**

Ingredients:

- ✓ Freshly ground black pepper.
- ✓ 2 tablespoons of balsamic vinegar
- ✓ 1 cup of raspberries

Directions:

- ❖ On four serving plates, make an equal layer of lettuce.
- ❖ Assemble the shallots and asparagus on top of the vegetables.

Ingredients:

- ✓ 1 shallot, both the green and white parts, sliced
- ✓ 1 cup asparagus, cut into long ribbons with a potato peeler
- ✓ 2 cups of shredded green lettuce
- ❖ On top of salads, place raspberries, distributing berries equally.
- ❖ Spoon with balsamic vinegar for salads.
- ❖ And season with a little black pepper.

185) Stir-fried chicken

Preparation Time: 3-4 min   **Cooking Time**: 10 min   **Servings: 4**

Ingredients:

- ✓ 3 cups of hot cooked rice
- ✓ 3 cups of frozen mixed vegetables
- ✓ 2 tablespoons of canola oil
- ✓ 1 ½ tablespoon of cornstarch

Directions:

- ❖ Wash and cut chicken into 1-inch pieces; set aside.
- ❖ Mix together the vinegar, honey, cornstarch, pineapple juice and soy sauce. Set this aside as well.
- ❖ In a large skillet, heat oil and sauté fresh vegetables until crisp-tender, about 3 minutes, then remove from heat.

Ingredients:

- ✓ 1 ½ tablespoons low-sodium soy sauce
- ✓ 3 tablespoons of pineapple juice
- ✓ 3 spoons of honey
- ✓ 3 tablespoons of vinegar
- ✓ 12 ounces of chicken breast, boneless and skinless
- ❖ On a hot griddle, cook the chicken for about 3 to 4 minutes and then transfer the chicken to a plate.
- ❖ Add your sauce and whisk until thick and bubbly.
- ❖ Return the vegetables and stir everything together.
- ❖ Cook the sauce for another minute or so and then serve it with rice.

186) Chicken and leek pie filling

Preparation Time: 15 min   **Cooking Time**: 30 min   **Servings: 4**

Ingredients:
- ✓ 1 packet of ready-made pasta
- ✓ 2 leeks coarsely chopped
- ✓ 500g (1lb 2oz) leftover roast chicken
- ✓ 3 tablespoons of single or heavy cream

Ingredients:
- ✓ 350 ml low-salt chicken broth
- ✓ 30g (1oz) plain flour
- ✓ 30g (1oz) unsalted butter

Directions:
- ❖ Preheat the oven to 180° C/350° F/Gas 4 (160° C fan).
- ❖ Melt the butter in a saucepan over medium heat and add a little flour. Stir until a lump forms, then for a few minutes, continue to cook and stir. To prevent lumps from forming, use a whisk to add the chicken broth a little at a time. Let the sauce simmer for a few minutes until all the broth is included, and continue stirring until it has thickened.

- ❖ Boil the leeks in another saucepan until soft and drain.
- ❖ In an ovenproof dish, mix the leeks, cream and chicken with your sauce and decant. Gently oil the sides of the dish and finish with your pasta recipe of choice. When using a pastry curl or fork through the sides and a little beaten egg is glazed in. Bake for about 30 minutes or until the surface is soft golden brown.

187) Cucumber, dill and cabbage salad with lemon dressing

Preparation Time: 25 minutes plus 1 hour to chill   **Cooking Time**: None   **Servings: 4**

Ingredients:
- ✓ 2 cups shredded green cabbage
- ✓ 1 English cucumber, thinly sliced
- ✓ ¼ teaspoon freshly ground black pepper
- ✓ 2 tablespoons finely chopped shallot, green part only

Ingredients:
- ✓ 2 tablespoons of chopped fresh dill
- ✓ 2 tablespoons granulated sugar
- ✓ ¼ cup freshly squeezed lemon juice
- ✓ ¼ cup heavy cream

Directions:
- ❖ Mix the lemon juice, cream, dill, sugar, shallot and pepper in a medium bowl until well combined.
- ❖ Simply toss the cucumber and cabbage together in a large pot.

- ❖ In refrigerator, place salad and chill for about 1 hour.
- ❖ Mix well before eating.

188)   Kedgeree

Preparation Time: 15-20 min   **Cooking Time**: 15 min   **Servings: 4**

Ingredients:

- ✓ ½ a lemon
- ✓ 4 hard-boiled eggs
- ✓ 400ml of low-salt chicken stock
- ✓ 400g (14oz) haddock fillets or poached smoked cod

Directions:

- ❖ In a large skillet, heat oil, add onion and sauté until softened. To cover the rice in the oil, apply the curry powder and rice and stir. Cover with an airtight lid or foil and simmer over low heat until most of the water has drained (about 10 minutes). Add the broth or water.

Ingredients:

- ✓ 2 teaspoons of curry powder
- ✓ 1 tablespoon vegetable or olive oil
- ✓ ½ onion finely sliced
- ✓ 200g (7oz) long grain rice
- ❖ Place the quartered fish and eggs on top of the rice and replace the lid until most of the water has been absorbed. Continue cooking for a few more minutes over low heat and then turn off the heat, leaving the covered rice, fish and eggs to steam for 5-10 minutes, allowing the fish to warm through the garnish. Drop the lid when time is up and bake the fish with a squeeze of lemon juice over the rice.

189)   Fish cake

Preparation Time: 15-20 min   **Cooking Time**: 15 min   **Servings: 4**

Ingredients:

- ✓ 20g cheddar cheese, finely grated
- ✓ About 75 ml of semi-skimmed milk
- ✓ 200g (7oz) cream cheese (garlic and herb flavor)
- ✓ 600g (1lb 3oz) fish cake mix, boneless
- ✓ 1 tablespoon of dried mixed herbs (or fresh if available)

Directions:

- ❖ In boiling water, cook potatoes and nacelle until tender.
- ❖ Meanwhile, in a large nonstick skillet, heat the liquid. Apply the herbs and onion and simmer gently until the onion is juicy but not browned.
- ❖ In skillet, place fish and heat until fish is just done. Attach cream cheese and stir over heat until cream cheese is melted and almost boiling.

Ingredients:

- ✓ 1 onion, finely chopped
- ✓ 1 tablespoon vegetable or olive oil
- ✓ 300g (11oz) of swede, peeled and cut into pieces
- ✓ 300g (11oz) potatoes, peeled and cut into pieces

- ❖ To get a good creamy sauce, gradually add the milk. If desired, season with pepper.
- ❖ Pour the fish mixture into a preheated baking dish. Drain and mash the hot turnip and potatoes. Use the fish mixture to finish it off. Sprinkle with grated cheese and set until cheese is melted and browned under a hot grill. Serve with seasonal vegetables.

190) Toad in the Hole

Preparation Time: 15-20 min   **Cooking Time**: 40-45 min   **Servings: 4**

Ingredients:
- ✓ 2 tablespoons vegetable or olive oil
- ✓ 8 sausages
- ✓ 3 sprigs of thyme, leaves only (optional)
- ✓ 300ml milk

Directions:
- ❖ Heat the oven to 425° F/Gas 7 to 220° C (200° C fan).
- ❖ Pour flour and whisk mustard powder into a large mixing bowl. In the center, create a well, crack in the egg and then pour in a splash of milk. Stir with a wooden spoon before you have a smooth batter in the well, constantly adding a little flour. Now apply a little more milk and combine until you have mixed both milk and flour.
- ❖ Now you can have a thick batter that has the consistency of double chocolate, with no lumps.

Ingredients:
- ✓ 1 egg
- ✓ ½ teaspoon of English mustard powder
- ✓ 100g (3½oz) plain flour

- ❖ Pour it into the pitcher you weighed the milk into, then stir in the thyme, if you're using it, to pour it in better later.
- ❖ Use scissors to cut the strings between the sausages, then drop them into a 20 x 30 cm baking dish. Apply a tablespoon of grease, toss the sausages to completely cover the bottom of the pan, and then bake for 15 minutes in the oven.
- ❖ Remove the hot tray from the oven and quickly add the batter. When it reaches hot fat, it may sizzle and bubble a bit. Return it to the oven, and then bake until the batter is cooked through, well risen and crispy, 40 minutes. It should look well cooked, not messy or runny, when you stick the tip of a knife into the batter in the center of the pan.

191) Pan-fried pork chop with creamy leek sauce

Preparation Time: 15 min   **Cooking Time**: 15 min   **Servings: 2**

Ingredients:
- ✓ 1 tablespoon fresh parsley, chopped
- ✓ 150 ml of heavy cream
- ✓ 50ml milk
- ✓ knob of unsalted butter
- ✓ 2 sprigs of thyme, leaves only

Directions:
- ❖ Heat a skillet or griddle until light. Brush the sliced pork with oil and return it to the skillet to cook for six minutes. Change the chop and cook for another six minutes or until cooked and browned. The juices may run clear as fried when pierced with a sharp knife.

Ingredients:
- ✓ ½ washed and sliced leek
- ✓ 1 garlic clove, peeled and chopped
- ✓ 1 tablespoon vegetable or olive oil
- ✓ 2 pork chops

- ❖ Remove from heat and set aside for three minutes to cool slightly.
- ❖ Heat the oil and butter in a leek pan and sauté the garlic with the leek and thyme leaves to soften for 3-4 minutes.
- ❖ Include the milk, cream and parsley, then reduce the heat and simmer for another 6-8 minutes gently, stirring regularly.
- ❖ Spoon over the pork chop with the creamy leek sauce and eat.

192) Tabbouleh

Preparation Time: 30 min plus 1 hour for refrigeration

Cooking Time: None

Servings: 6

Ingredients:
- ✓ Freshly ground black pepper.
- ✓ Zest of 1 lemon
- ✓ Juice of 1 lemon
- ✓ 2 tablespoons of olive oil
- ✓ ¼ cup finely chopped fresh cilantro
- ✓ ¼ cup finely chopped fresh parsley

Ingredients:
- ✓ 1 cup chopped eggplant, boiled until tender
- ✓ ½ zucchini, finely chopped, boiled until tender
- ✓ ½ yellow bell pepper, boiled and chopped
- ✓ ½ red bell pepper, boiled and finely chopped
- ✓ 4 cups of cooked white rice

Directions:
- ❖ Mix the red bell bell pepper, rice, yellow bell bell pepper, eggplant, zucchini, parsley, cilantro, lemon juice, olive oil and lemon zest in a large bowl until well mixed.

- ❖ Add a little black pepper for seasoning.
- ❖ Before serving, chill the salad in the refrigerator for at least 1 hour.

193) Jars of eggs and vegetables for microwave

Preparation Time: 5 min

Cooking Time: 5 min

Servings: 4

Ingredients:
- ✓ 8 big eggs
- ✓ 1/4 cup mushrooms
- ✓ 1/4 cup broccoli
- ✓ 1/4 cup onion
- ✓ 1/4 cup of bell bell pepper

Ingredients:
- ✓ 4 tablespoons shredded natural cheddar cheese
- ✓ 8 ounces of turkey sausage
- ✓ 1 fresh jalapeño bell pepper (optional)
- ✓ 4 microwaveable jars with lids

Directions:
- ❖ Heat turkey sausage in a small skillet until browned. While frying, cut it into crumbs.
- ❖ Through the interior coating with cooking spray, prepare the jars.
- ❖ Dice the cabbage, broccoli, mushrooms and bell bell pepper. Combine the sliced vegetables in a shallow bowl. Cut in the jalapeño pepper.
- ❖ In each pot, add 1/4 cup bacon, 1 tablespoon cheese, 1/4 cup diced vegetable mixture and 2 or 3 slices jalapeño bell pepper.

- ❖ Cover and store jars in the refrigerator for up to 4 days.
- ❖ Beat the two eggs, apply them to the container and mix well until you are about to feed. Stir in the microwave for 30 seconds. Repeat before setting up the chickens. (Depending on your microwave, this may take 1-1/2 to 2 minutes).
- ❖ Gently remove the container from the microwave and enjoy.

194) Strawberry chia overnight oats

Preparation Time: 10 min

Cooking Time: None

Servings: 1

Ingredients:
- ✓ 5 medium strawberries
- ✓ 2/3 cup of unsweetened almond milk
- ✓ 1 tablespoon chia seeds

Ingredients:
- ✓ 1/2 scoop of vanilla whey protein powder (optional)
- ✓ 1/2 cup old-fashioned rolled oats, dry
- ❖ Overnight, place in the refrigerator.
- ❖ Cut up strawberries before eating and add to oats. When needed, add the sugar substitute of preference.

Directions:
- ❖ Mix together the protein powder, oats, chia seeds and almond milk in a medium bowl until well blended.
- ❖ through the oat mixture into an 8-12 ounce jar.

195)   Peanut and oat bars without cooking

Preparation Time: 10 min   **Cooking Time**: 1 hour   **Servings: 10**

Ingredients:
- ✓ 1/4 cup mini chocolate chips
- ✓ 1/3 cup agave nectar
- ✓ 1/2 cup of peanut butter
- ✓ 1/2 cup of whey protein powder

Directions:
- ❖ Line a 5 x 7-inch or 8-inch square baking pan with greaseproof paper or parchment.
- ❖ Mix the oatmeal, cinnamon and salt in a medium bowl.
- ❖ Mix protein powder, peanut butter and agave nectar in a medium bowl; whisk until smooth.
- ❖ Mix peanut butter mixture with oats until completely blended.

Ingredients:
- ✓ 1/8 teaspoon salt
- ✓ 1/2 teaspoon of cinnamon
- ✓ 2 cups rolled oats, dry

- ❖ Evenly mix Pat into lined baking dish. Sprinkle in chocolate chips and pat evenly. For at least 1 hour, refrigerate.
- ❖ To make the 10 bars divide into five pieces, then into halves. Cover each bar in plastic wrap, if necessary. Keep in refrigerator until you are going to consume or on-the-go.

196)   Tortilla Beef Rollup Lunch Box

Preparation Time: 10 min   **Cooking Time**: None   **Servings: 1**

Ingredients:
- ✓ 10 unsalted almonds
- ✓ 1/2 cup of grapes
- ✓ 1/2 teaspoon of herb seasoning mix
- ✓ 1 tablespoon whipped cream cheese
- ✓ 1 6-inch flour tortilla

Directions:
- ❖ Slice beef and cucumber with roast; chop onion and bell bell pepper. Remove the rib from the romaine lettuce leaf.
- ❖ Spread cream cheese on tortilla to make a beef roll-up. Layer the top with roast beef strips and vegetables. Sprinkle with spices.

Ingredients:
- ✓ 1 leaf of romaine lettuce
- ✓ 1/4 red onion red bell pepper
- ✓ 1 slice
- ✓ 4 cucumbers
- ✓ 2-1/2 ounces of cooked roast beef

- ❖ Roll up the tortilla like a jelly roll and break it into four sections.
- ❖ Place the roll-up, grapes and almonds on a plate or in a divided lunch jar.

197)   All American Meatloaf

Preparation Time: 15 min   **Cooking Time**: 50 min   **Servings**: 6

Ingredients:

- ✓ 1 tablespoon water
- ✓ 1/2 teaspoon apple cider vinegar
- ✓ 1 tablespoon of brown sugar
- ✓ 1/3 cup of ketchup
- ✓ 1/4 teaspoon of black pepper

Directions:

- ❖ Preheat the oven to about 350° F.
- ❖ Place crackers and crush with a rolling pin in a large zipper pocket. Finely chop onions.
- ❖ Lightly brush a loaf pan with nonstick cooking oil.
- ❖ Combine crushed crackers, cabbage, ground beef, cheese, milk and black pepper in a large dish. Mix thoroughly.

Ingredients:

- ✓ 2 tablespoons of 1% low-fat milk
- ✓ 1 large egg
- ✓ 1 pound of lean beef (10% fat)
- ✓ 2 tablespoons of onion
- ✓ 20 squares of salted crackers, unsalted tops
- ❖ Move the mixture to the loaf pan. For 40 minutes, roast.
- ❖ Mix ketchup, brown sugar, vinegar and water in a small bowl to create a dressing.
- ❖ Remove fried meatloaf from oven and coat with sauce.
- ❖ Return the pan to the oven and bake for 10 minutes or until the internal temperature is above 160 degrees F.
- ❖ Cut and serve into 6 pieces.

198)   Quick pan-fried chicken

Preparation Time: 10 min   **Cooking Time**: 10 min   **Servings**: 4

Ingredients:

- ✓ 2 tablespoons of dried basil
- ✓ 2 spoons of honey
- ✓ 2 tablespoons of balsamic vinegar

Directions:

- ❖ Heat olive oil over medium heat in a skillet. Sprinkle with pepper and toss with chicken.
- ❖ Fry the chicken on both sides for 5 minutes, until golden brown.
- ❖ Add the balsamic vinegar and sauté, turning the chicken to cover, for one minute.

Ingredients:

- ✓ 1/4 teaspoon of black pepper
- ✓ 1 pound boneless, skinless chicken breasts
- ✓ 2 tablespoons of olive oil
- ❖ Apply the basil and honey. Stir and turn to cover the chicken. Cook longer for 1 minute.
- ❖ Mix the sauce in a dish and pour over the chicken.

199)   Pilaf rice better than packaged rice

Preparation Time: 10 min   **Cooking Time**: 25 min   **Servings**: 6

Ingredients:

- ✓ 1 tablespoon of chicken broth granules
- ✓ 1 cup parboiled rice, uncooked
- ✓ 2 ounces of vermicelli noodles, uncooked

Directions:

- ❖ Melt 1 tablespoon butter over medium-high heat in a skillet.
- ❖ Divide vermicelli into 2-inch portions and cook until noodles begin to brown, stirring regularly.
- ❖ Substitute the leftover rice and butter. Stir to combine.

Ingredients:

- ✓ 2 cups of water
- ✓ 2 tablespoons unsalted butter
- ✓ 1 tablespoon onion and herb seasoning mix
- ❖ In the skillet, apply the chicken bouillon granules, water and herb seasoning. To mix ingredients, whisk.
- ❖ Cover and bring to a boil. Lower the heat and simmer for 20 minutes. Do not remove the lid.
- ❖ Turn off the heat and prepare for another 5 minutes to stay covered.
- ❖ Flatten and serve with a fork.

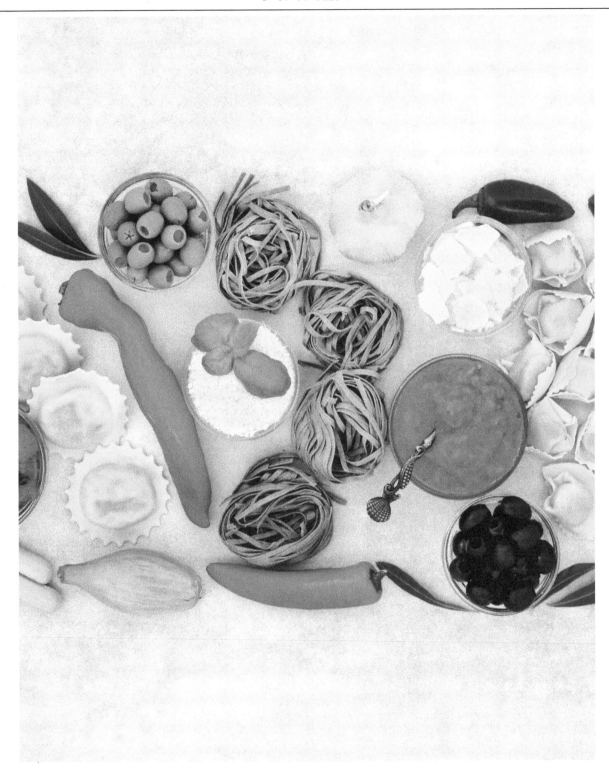

200)   Beefsteak chunks

Preparation Time: 10 minutes   **Cooking Time**: 40 minutes   **Servings: 4**

Ingredients:

- ✓ 1 lb. beef steak, diced
- ✓ 1 tablespoon of olive oil

Directions:

- ❖ In mixing bowl, mix meat with olive oil, dried dill and dried basil.
- ❖ Place the spiced meat in the tray in one layer.

Ingredients:

- ✓ 1 teaspoon of dried dill
- ✓ ½ teaspoon of dried basil
- ❖ Then transfer the tray to the preheated 365F oven and bake for 40 minutes. Stir the meat occasionally to avoid burning it.

201)   Bowl of ground beef

Preparation Time: 10 minutes   **Cooking Time**: 20 minutes   **Servings: 4**

Ingredients:

- ✓ 1 tablespoon of dried parsley
- ✓ ½ teaspoon of dried basil
- ✓ 1 tablespoon of olive oil

Directions:

- ❖ Pour the olive oil into the casserole dish.
- ❖ Add the beef tenderloin and lime juice. Carefully stir the meat and cook over medium heat for 10 minutes.

Ingredients:

- ✓ 1 tablespoon of lime juice
- ✓ 12 ounces of beef tenderloin, minced

- ❖ Then add all the remaining ingredients and mix thoroughly.
- ❖ Close the lid and cook the meat over medium heat for another 10 minutes.

202)   Meatloaf with basil

Preparation Time: 10 minutes   **Cooking Time**: 40 minutes   **Servings: 4**

Ingredients:

- ✓ 1 tablespoon of dried basil
- ✓ 2 egg whites, beaten

Directions:

- ❖ Brush the loaf mold with olive oil from the inside.
- ❖ Then mix the basil with the egg whites and beef tenderloin.

Ingredients:

- ✓ 10 ounces of beef tenderloin, minced
- ✓ 1 teaspoon of olive oil
- ❖ When the mixture is smooth, transfer it to the loaf mold and flatten it well.
- ❖ Bake the meatloaf at 360F for 40 minutes.
- ❖ Then cool the meal well and slice.

203)   Sirloin of beef with rosemary

Preparation Time: 10 minutes   **Cooking Time**: 30 minutes   **Servings: 4**

Ingredients:

- ✓ 1 tablespoon of dried rosemary
- ✓ 1 pound of beef sirloin

Directions:

- ❖ Rub the beef sirloin with dried rosemary and drizzle with olive oil.

Ingredients:

- ✓ 1 teaspoon of olive oil

- ❖ Then place the meat in the tray.
- ❖ Cook beef at 360F for 15 minutes per side.

204)   Stuffed beef meatloaf

Preparation Time: 10 minutes   **Cooking Time**: 40 minutes   **Servings: 4**

Ingredients:

- ✓ 1 carrot, peeled, coarsely chopped
- ✓ 10 ounces of beef tenderloin, minced
- ✓ ½ chopped onion

Directions:

- ❖ In mixing bowl, mix beef tenderloin, chopped onion and ground paprika.
- ❖ Then brush the loaf mold with olive oil from the inside.

Ingredients:

- ✓ 1 teaspoon ground paprika
- ✓ 1 teaspoon of olive oil

- ❖ Place the meat mixture in the loaf mold and flatten well.
- ❖ Place the shredded carrot inside the patty.
- ❖ Bake the meatloaf at 360F for 40 minutes.

205)   Beef with sage

Preparation Time: 10 minutes   **Cooking Time**: 45 minutes   **Servings: 4**

Ingredients:

- ✓ 1 teaspoon of dried sage
- ✓ ½ teaspoon of dried oregano

Directions:

- ❖ Mix meat with sage, oregano and ground turmeric.
- ❖ Place the meat in the aluminum foil.

Ingredients:

- ✓ ½ teaspoon ground turmeric
- ✓ 1 lb beef tenderloin
- ❖ Then transfer the meat to the preheated 360F oven and bake for 45 minutes.
- ❖ Remove the foil from the cooked meat and slice it.

206)   Ginger beef

Preparation Time: 10 minutes   **Cooking Time**: 14 minutes   **Servings: 4**

Ingredients:

- ✓ 1 teaspoon ground ginger
- ✓ 1 teaspoon of olive oil

Directions:

- ❖ Rub the beef sirloin with ground ginger and olive oil.

Ingredients:

- ✓ 1 pound of beef sirloin

- ❖ Then preheat the grill to 400F.
- ❖ Place the meat in the grill and cook for 7 minutes per side.

207)   Tender beef with cinnamon

Preparation Time: 10 minutes   **Cooking Time**: 40 minutes   **Servings: 4**

Ingredients:

- ✓ 1 tablespoon of lime juice
- ✓ ½ teaspoon ground cinnamon

Directions:

- ❖ Rub beef with ground cinnamon and sprinkle with lime juice and olive oil.
- ❖ Wrap the meat in plastic wrap.

Ingredients:

- ✓ 1 lb beef tenderloin
- ✓ 1 tablespoon of olive oil
- ❖ Bake the wrapped meat for 40 minutes at 365F.
- ❖ Then allow the meat to rest for 10 minutes.
- ❖ Remove the meat from the sheet and slice it.

208) Beef with onion

Preparation Time: 10 minutes   **Cooking Time**: 50 minutes   **Servings: 4**

Ingredients:

- ✓ 1 onion, sliced
- ✓ 1 tablespoon of olive oil

Directions:

- ❖ Brush the baking sheet with olive oil.
- ❖ Then slice the beef tenderloin and mix it with the chili flakes.

Ingredients:

- ✓ 1 teaspoon of chili flakes
- ✓ 1 lb beef tenderloin
- ❖ Place the beef in the baking dish in one layer and cover with the sliced onion.
- ❖ Cover the pan with aluminum foil and bake the meat at 360F for 50 minutes.

209) Bell pepper and beef sauce

Preparation Time: 10 minutes   **Cooking Time**: 45 minutes   **Servings: 4**

Ingredients:

- ✓ 1 cup bell bell pepper, chopped
- ✓ ½ chili pepper, chopped
- ✓ 6 ounces of beef tenderloin, minced

Directions:

- ❖ Place all ingredients in the saucepan and stir gently.

Ingredients:

- ✓ ½ cup of water
- ✓ 1 teaspoon ground nutmeg

- ❖ Close the lid and cook the sauté over medium heat for 45 minutes. Stir occasionally to avoid burning.

210) Beef with paprika

Preparation Time: 10 minutes   **Cooking Time**: 55 minutes   **Servings: 4**

Ingredients:

- ✓ 1 tablespoon ground paprika
- ✓ 1 tablespoon of olive oil

Directions:

- ❖ Mix the lime juice with the olive oil and ground paprika.
- ❖ Then brush the beef tenderloin with the paprika mixture and wrap it in foil.

Ingredients:

- ✓ 2 tablespoons of lime juice
- ✓ 1 lb beef tenderloin
- ❖ Bake the meat at 360F for 55 minutes.
- ❖ Then remove the foil from the beef and slice it into portions.

211) Sirloin of beef with tender shallots

Preparation Time: 5 minutes   **Cooking Time**: 60 minutes   **Servings: 4**

Ingredients:

- ✓ 1 pound of beef sirloin
- ✓ 2 ounces shallot, chopped

Directions:

- ❖ Slice the beef loin and place in the casserole dish.
- ❖ Add the rice milk and cook the meat over medium-low heat for 55 minutes.

Ingredients:

- ✓ ½ cup of rice milk

- ❖ After this, add the scallions and cook the meat for another 5 minutes.

212) Sautéed beef and onion

Preparation Time: 10 minutes   **Cooking Time**: 45 minutes   **Servings: 4**

Ingredients:
- ✓ 1 large onion, sliced
- ✓ 1 garlic clove, peeled

Directions:
- ❖ Cut the beef loin and place in the skillet.
- ❖ Roast it for 2-3 minutes.

Ingredients:
- ✓ 1 pound of beef sirloin
- ✓ 1 cup of water
- ❖ Then stir in the meat and add the onion. Carefully mix the ingredients together and add the water.
- ❖ Close the lid and cook the saute over medium heat for 40 minutes.

213) Carrot meatballs

Preparation Time: 15 minutes   **Cooking Time**: 30 minutes   **Servings: 4**

Ingredients:
- ✓ ¼ cup carrot, grated
- ✓ 7 ounces of ground beef sirloin
- ✓ ½ teaspoon ground nutmeg

Directions:
- ❖ In the bowl, mix the carrot with the sirloin, nutmeg and ground cilantro.
- ❖ Make meatballs with the meat mixture.

Ingredients:
- ✓ ½ teaspoon of ground coriander
- ✓ 1 teaspoon of olive oil
- ❖ After this, brush the casserole mold with olive oil.
- ❖ Place the patties in the casserole dish and cover with aluminum foil.
- ❖ Bake the meatballs at 360F for 30 minutes.

214) Cumin seeds Beef

Preparation Time: 10 minutes   **Cooking Time**: 30 minutes   **Servings: 4**

Ingredients:
- ✓ 1 teaspoon of cumin seeds
- ✓ 1 lb. beef tenderloin, sliced

Directions:
- ❖ Preheat the pan well.
- ❖ Add the cumin seeds and toast them for 1 minute.
- ❖ Then add the olive oil and sliced beef.

Ingredients:
- ✓ 1 tablespoon of olive oil
- ✓ 2 tablespoons water
- ❖ Roast the meat for 4 minutes per side.
- ❖ Add the water and close the lid.
- ❖ Simmer the beef over medium heat for an additional 20 minutes.

215) Beef ribs masala

Preparation Time: 10 minutes   **Cooking Time**: 30 minutes   **Servings: 4**

Ingredients:
- ✓ 1 lb beef ribs
- ✓ 1 tablespoon of garam masala

Directions:
- ❖ Mix the garam masala with the rice milk and pour into the saucepan.

Ingredients:
- ✓ ½ cup of rice milk
- ❖ Add the beef chops and close the lid.
- ❖ Cook the meat over medium heat for 30 minutes.

216)   Spiced Roast Beef

Preparation Time: 10 minutes   **Cooking Time**: 40 minutes   **Servings: 4**

Ingredients:

- ✓   1 teaspoon of ground coriander
- ✓   ½ teaspoon of dried thyme
- ✓   ½ teaspoon of dried oregano

Directions:

- ❖   Rub the beef loin with ground cilantro, dried thyme, oregano, chili powder and canola oil.
- ❖   Then place the beef in the baking dish.

Ingredients:

- ✓   ¼ teaspoon of chili powder
- ✓   1 tablespoon of canola oil
- ✓   Loin of beef 1 pound
- ❖   Transfer the pan to the preheated 360F oven and bake for 40 minutes.
- ❖   Cut hot milk into portions.

217)   **Beef Fajita**

Preparation Time: 10 minutes   **Cooking Time**: 20 minutes   **Servings: 4**

Ingredients:

- ✓   1 tablespoon of Fajita seasonings
- ✓   1 tablespoon of olive oil

Directions:

- ❖   Preheat the olive oil in the skillet.
- ❖   Add the beef loin and fajita seasonings. Mix ingredients together well.

Ingredients:

- ✓   1 lb. beef loin, cut into strips
- ❖   Close the lid and cook the beef over medium heat for 10 minutes.
- ❖   After this, mix the meat well and cook it for another 10 minutes.

218)   **Ground beef with shallots**

Preparation Time: 5 minutes   **Cooking Time**: 20 minutes   **Servings: 4**

Ingredients:

- ✓   3 ounces shallots, chopped
- ✓   10 ounces of beef loin, minced

Directions:

- ❖   Mix the beef loin with the ground cilantro and place the mixture in the casserole dish.
- ❖   Roast for 2-3 minutes over medium heat.

Ingredients:

- ✓   1 tablespoon of rice milk
- ✓   ½ teaspoon of ground coriander
- ❖   After this, add the rice milk and scallions.
- ❖   Close the lid and cook the meal over medium heat for another 15 minutes.

219)   **Corned beef**

Preparation Time: 10 minutes   **Cooking Time**: 65 minutes   **Servings: 4**

Ingredients:

- ✓   1 teaspoon of spices
- ✓   1 teaspoon of pepper
- ✓   1 cinnamon stick

Directions:

- ❖   Place all ingredients in the saucepan and close the lid.

Ingredients:

- ✓   Loin of beef 1 pound
- ✓   3 cups of water
- ✓   2 tablespoons of lime juice
- ❖   Cook the meat over medium heat for 65 minutes.
- ❖   Then allow the meat to rest for 10 minutes.

220) Indian style beef loin

Preparation Time: 10 minutes   **Cooking Time**: 25 minutes   **Servings: 4**

Ingredients:
- ✓ Loin of beef 1 pound
- ✓ ½ teaspoon of curry powder
- ✓ ½ teaspoon of garam masala

Directions:
- ❖ Rub the beef loin with curry powder and garam masala.
- ❖ Then preheat the pan well and add the olive oil.

Ingredients:
- ✓ 1 tablespoon of olive oil
- ✓ ½ cup of rice milk

- ❖ Place beef in hot oil and roast for 5 minutes per side over medium heat.
- ❖ Add the rice milk and close the lid.
- ❖ Cook the beef over medium heat for an additional 15 minutes.

221) Hungarian goulash

Preparation Time: 5 minutes   **Cooking Time**: 55 minutes   **Servings: 4**

Ingredients:
- ✓ 2 carrots, peeled, chopped
- ✓ 1 oz shallot, chopped
- ✓ 10 ounces of beef tenderloin, minced

Directions:
- ❖ Place all ingredients in the saucepan and stir gently.

Ingredients:
- ✓ 1 cup of water
- ✓ 1 onion, diced
- ✓ 1 teaspoon of dried rosemary
- ❖ Close the lid and cook the goulash over medium-low heat for 55 minutes.
- ❖ When all the goulash ingredients are tender, the meal is cooked.

222) Saffron meatballs dinner

Preparation Time: 15 minutes   **Cooking Time**: 10 minutes   **Servings: 4**

Ingredients:
- ✓ ¼ teaspoon of dry saffron
- ✓ 10 ounces of beef loin, minced

Directions:
- ❖ Pour the olive oil into the pan and preheat well.
- ❖ Meanwhile, mix the beef loin with the minced garlic and saffron.

Ingredients:
- ✓ ½ teaspoon of minced garlic
- ✓ 1 teaspoon of olive oil

- ❖ Make small patties from the meat mixture and place them in the hot oil.
- ❖ Roast the meatballs for 4 minutes per side.

223) Minced beef casserole

Preparation Time: 10 minutes   **Cooking Time**: 35 minutes   **Servings: 6**

Ingredients:

- ✓ 8 ounces of beef loin, minced
- ✓ ½ onion, diced
- ✓ 1 cup cauliflower, chopped

Directions:

- ❖ Mix the beef loin with the diced onion and Parmesan cheese.
- ❖ Place the mixture in the casserole mold and flatten well.

Ingredients:

- ✓ ½ cup of rice milk
- ✓ 1 oz Parmesan cheese, grated

- ❖ Top with the cauliflower and cover with aluminum foil.
- ❖ Cook the casserole over medium heat for 35 minutes.

224) Beef soffritto and Portobello

Preparation Time: 10 minutes   **Cooking Time**: 35 minutes   **Servings: 4**

Ingredients:

- ✓ 2 Portobello mushrooms, chopped
- ✓ 8 ounces of beef tenderloin, minced
- ✓ 1 tablespoon of olive oil

Directions:

- ❖ Pour the olive oil into the saucepan and preheat well.
- ❖ Add the beef tenderloin and roast for 3-4 minutes.

Ingredients:

- ✓ ½ onion, diced
- ✓ 1 cup of water
- ✓ 1 teaspoon of chili powder
- ❖ Then mix the meat well and add the mushrooms.
- ❖ Add the onion, chili powder and water.
- ❖ Close the lid.
- ❖ Cook the saute over medium heat for 30 minutes.

225) Boiled beef with sauce

Preparation Time: 25 minutes   **Cooking Time**: 40 minutes   **Servings: 4**

Ingredients:

- ✓ 12 ounces beef tenderloin, coarsely chopped
- ✓ 2 cups of water
- ✓ ¼ cup of rice milk
- ✓ 1 teaspoon of white flour

Directions:

- ❖ Pour the water into the saucepan.
- ❖ Add the beef and cook for 40 minutes.
- ❖ Meanwhile, mix the rice milk with the white flour, ground nutmeg and cardamom.

Ingredients:

- ✓ 1 teaspoon ground nutmeg
- ✓ ¼ teaspoon ground cardamom
- ✓ ½ teaspoon of curry powder

- ❖ Add the curry powder.
- ❖ Stir the mixture until smooth.
- ❖ Bring the liquid to a boil and remove from heat.
- ❖ When beef is cooked, transfer to bowls and cover with rice milk sauce.

226)   Beef with tarragon

Preparation Time: 10 minutes   **Cooking Time**: 40 minutes   **Servings: 4**

Ingredients:
- ✓   1 teaspoon of dried tarragon
- ✓   1 lb beef tenderloin

Directions:
- ❖   Mix beef tenderloin with tarragon and olive oil.

Ingredients:
- ✓   1 tablespoon of olive oil

- ❖   Then wrap the meat in plastic wrap.
- ❖   Cook the beef at 365F for 40 minutes.

227)   Rolls of arugula and beef

Preparation Time: 20 minutes   **Cooking Time**: 10 minutes   **Servings: 4**

Ingredients:
- ✓   8 ounces of beef loin, boiled, shredded
- ✓   2 cups of arugula
- ✓   ½ carrot, grated

Directions:
- ❖   Mix the beef with the grated carrot and chili.
- ❖   Then place the beef mixture on the arugula leaves and roll them up.

Ingredients:
- ✓   ½ cup of water
- ✓   1 hot pepper, diced

- ❖   Place the rolls in the casserole dish, add the water.
- ❖   Close the lid and cook the rolls over medium heat for 10 minutes.

228)   Roast beef with oregano

Preparation Time: 10 minutes   **Cooking Time**: 20 minutes   **Servings: 4**

Ingredients:
- ✓   1 lb roast beef
- ✓   1 tablespoon of dried oregano

Directions:
- ❖   Preheat the olive oil in the skillet well.
- ❖   Mix the oregano with the roast beef.

Ingredients:
- ✓   1 tablespoon of olive oil

- ❖   Place the meat in the hot oil and roast for 10 minutes per side over medium heat.

229)   Grilled beef sirloin with carrots

Preparation Time: 10 minutes   **Cooking Time**: 10 minutes   **Servings: 4**

Ingredients:
- ✓   1 pound of beef loin, cut into strips
- ✓   1 teaspoon of dried dill

Directions:
- ❖   Mix beef loin with olive oil and dried dill.
- ❖   Then preheat the grill to 400F.

Ingredients:
- ✓   1 carrot, cut into strips
- ✓   1 tablespoon of olive oil
- ❖   Place the beef and carrot in the grill.
- ❖   Cook the meal for 4 minutes per side.

230)   Veal rolls with basil

Preparation Time: 10 minutes   **Cooking Time**: 35 minutes   **Servings: 4**

Ingredients:

- ✓ 1 tablespoon of dried basil
- ✓ 1 onion, sliced

Directions:

- ❖ Cut the veal into 4 portions,
- ❖ Then rub the meat with dried basil.

Ingredients:

- ✓ Fillet of veal 1 pound
- ✓ 1 teaspoon of canola oil
- ❖ Spread the onion over the fillets and roll them up.
- ❖ Place the meat rolls in the tray and drizzle with canola oil.
- ❖ Bake the meat rolls at 360F for 35 minutes.

231)   Mouth watering beef chunks

Preparation Time: 10 minutes   **Cooking Time**: 40 minutes   **Servings: 4**

Ingredients:

- ✓ 1 teaspoon ground turmeric
- ✓ 1 garlic clove, peeled

Directions:

- ❖ Place all ingredients in the casserole dish.
- ❖ Gently stir the mixture and close the lid.

Ingredients:

- ✓ 1 lb. beef loin, diced
- ✓ ½ cup of rice milk
- ❖ Simmer the flour over medium heat for 40 minutes. Stir occasionally to avoid burning.

232)   Soft goulash

Preparation Time: 10 minutes   **Cooking Time**: 50 minutes   **Servings: 4**

Ingredients:

- ✓ 1 pound of beef tenderloin, minced
- ✓ 2 garlic cloves, peeled
- ✓ ½ teaspoon ground clove

Directions:

- ❖ Rub the beef tenderloin with the ground clove and cardamom.
- ❖ Place the meat in the casserole dish.

Ingredients:

- ✓ ¼ teaspoon ground cardamom
- ✓ 2 onions, diced
- ✓ 1 cup of water
- ❖ Add all remaining ingredients and close the lid.
- ❖ Cook the goulash over medium heat for 50 minutes.

233)   Steak chunks with cayenne pepper

Preparation Time: 10 minutes   **Cooking Time**: 24 minutes   **Servings: 4**

Ingredients:

- ✓ 1 lb beefsteak
- ✓ 1 teaspoon of cayenne pepper

Directions:

- ❖ Rub the flank steak with cayenne pepper and cut into bites.

Ingredients:

- ✓ 1 teaspoon of olive oil
- ❖ Then drizzle the meat with olive oil and place it in the tray in one layer.
- ❖ Bake the meat at 360F for 12 minutes per side.

234)   Beef brussels sprouts

Preparation Time: 5 minutes   **Cooking Time**: 40 minutes   **Servings: 4**

Ingredients:

- ✓ 1 cup Brussels sprouts, chopped
- ✓ 12 ounces of beef sirloin, minced
- ✓ 1 cup of water

Directions:

- ❖ Place all ingredients in the saucepan and mix well.

Ingredients:

- ✓ 1 teaspoon of peppercorns
- ✓ 1 teaspoon ground paprika
- ✓ 1 teaspoon of dried basil
- ❖ Close the lid and cook the beef over medium heat for 40 minutes or until the beef is tender.

235)   Beef with cauliflower

Preparation Time: 10 minutes   **Cooking Time**: 50 minutes   **Servings: 4**

Ingredients:

- ✓ 1 cup cauliflower, chopped
- ✓ 12 ounces of beef tenderloin, minced
- ✓ 1 clove of garlic, diced

Directions:

- ❖ Mix beef with dried thyme and diced garlic.
- ❖ Place the beef in the casserole dish and add the water.

Ingredients:

- ✓ 1 cup of water
- ✓ 1 teaspoon of dried thyme

- ❖ Add the cauliflower and close the lid.
- ❖ Cook beef over medium heat for 50 minutes. Stir occasionally.

236)   Beef Stroganoff without mushrooms

Preparation Time: 10 minutes   **Cooking Time**: 30 minutes   **Servings: 4**

Ingredients:

- ✓ 12 ounces of sirloin steak, cut into strips
- ✓ 1 tablespoon of olive oil
- ✓ 1 cup of water
- ✓ 1 teaspoon of white flour

Directions:

- ❖ Pour the olive oil into the casserole dish and preheat it.
- ❖ Add the beefsteak and minced garlic.
- ❖ Roast the meat for 2 minutes per side.
- ❖ After this, add the onion, water and rice milk.

Ingredients:

- ✓ 1 teaspoon of minced garlic
- ✓ ¼ cup of rice milk
- ✓ 1 onion, sliced

- ❖ Stir the mixture and bring it to a boil. Simmer the meat for 10 minutes.
- ❖ Then add the white flour and mix in the flour until smooth.
- ❖ Close the lid and cook the meat for another 5 minutes.

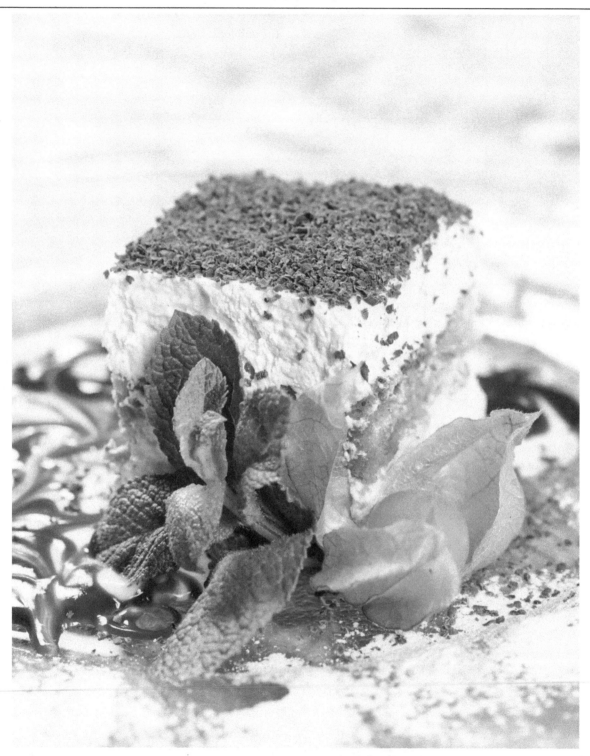

Preparation Time: 5 minutes   **Cooking Time**: 5 minutes   **Servings: 1**

Ingredients:
- ✓ 1/4 teaspoon of cinnamon
- ✓ 1/2 cup of almond milk
- ✓ 1 large egg

Ingredients:
- ✓ 1/3 cup quick-cooking oatmeal
- ✓ 1/2 medium apple

Directions:
- ❖ Twist and coarsely cut apple halves.
- ❖ In a large bowl, mix the egg, oatmeal and almond milk. Using a fork, mix well. Add the apple and cinnamon. When well combined, mix again.

- ❖ Cook in microwave for 2 minutes, on high heat. With a fork, fluff up. If necessary, cook for an additional 30-60 seconds.
- ❖ If thinner cereal is needed, add a little more milk or water

238) **Lemon and lime sorbet**

Preparation Time: 5 min plus 3 hours cooling time   **Cooking Time**: 15 minutes   **Servings: 8**

Ingredients:
- ✓ ½ cup heavy cream (whipping cream)
- ✓ Juice of 1 lime
- ✓ Zest of 1 lime
- ✓ ½ cup of freshly squeezed lemon juice

Ingredients:
- ✓ 3 tablespoons of lemon zest, divided
- ✓ 1 cup granulated sugar
- ✓ 2 cups of water

Directions:
- ❖ Over medium-high heat, place a large saucepan and add the water, sugar and two tablespoons of lemon zest.
- ❖ Bring the mixture to a boil and then reduce the heat for 15 minutes and simmer.

- ❖ Place the mixture in a large bowl and apply a tablespoon of lemon zest, lemon juice, lime zest and lime juice to the remaining mixture.
- ❖ Chill the mixture in the refrigerator for about 3 hours before it is absolutely cold.
- ❖ Blend and strain the mixture into an ice cream maker with the heavy cream.
- ❖ Freeze according to supplier's directions.

239) **Cherry Pie**

Preparation Time: 10-20 minutes   **Cooking Time**: 45 minutes   **Servings: 24**

Ingredients:
- ✓ 20 ounces of pie filling - cherry
- ✓ 1 teaspoon of baking soda
- ✓ 1 teaspoon baking powder
- ✓ 1 teaspoon of vanilla
- ✓ 2 cups of white flour

Ingredients:
- ✓ 1 cup of sour cream
- ✓ 1 cup of sugar
- ✓ 2 eggs
- ✓ ½ cup unsalted butter

Directions:
- ❖ Preheat the oven to about 350°F and, at room temperature, soften the butter
- ❖ Cream the eggs, sugar, vanilla and sour cream together,
- ❖ Combine baking powder, flour, and baking soda in another dish.

- ❖ Gradually mix the dry ingredients into the wet cream mixture, folding to mix completely. Grease a 9' x 13' baking dish and place the batter in it.
- ❖ Layer the cherry mixture equally over the batter.
- ❖ Bake for about 40 minutes, until golden brown.

240)   Sponge pudding with syrup

Preparation Time: 15-20 minutes   **Cooking Time**: 35-40 minutes   **Servings: 4**

Ingredients:

- ✓ 6 spoons of golden syrup
- ✓ 100g (3½oz) self-raising flour
- ✓ 2 eggs

Directions:

- ❖ In a saucepan or food processor, cream the butter and sugar.
- ❖ To prevent curdling, apply one egg and gently combine with one tablespoon of flour. Add the other egg and combine thoroughly.
- ❖ Fold the flour.

Ingredients:

- ✓ 100g (3½oz) caster sugar
- ✓ 100g (3½oz) softened unsalted butter

- ❖ Measure sugar into a buttered pudding bowl. On top of sugar, spoon cake mixture.
- ❖ With a fold, cover with a buttered sheet to allow for expansion.
- ❖ Bake for 35-40 minutes at 200°C (180°C fan)/400°F/Gas 6 until a skewer comes out clean.

241)   Crunchy apple granita

Preparation Time: 15 minutes plus 4 hours freezing time   **Cooking Time**:   **Servings: 4**

Ingredients:

- ✓ ¼ cup freshly squeezed lemon juice
- ✓ 2 cups unsweetened apple juice

Directions:

- ❖ Heat the sugar and water in a medium-sized saucepan over medium-high heat.
- ❖ Bring the mixture to a boil and then reduce the heat to low and simmer for about 15 more minutes or until the liquid has reduced by half.
- ❖ Remove the pan from the heat and pour the liquid into a large, shallow metal pan.

Ingredients:

- ✓ ½ cup of water
- ✓ ½ cup granulated sugar

- ❖ For about 30 minutes, let the mixture set and then stir in the apple juice and lemon juice.
- ❖ In a freezer, place your pan.
- ❖ Run a fork through the liquid after 1 hour to break up any ice crystals that have developed. Scrape down the sides as well.
- ❖ Return the pan to the freezer and continue to stir and scrape, making the slush every 20 minutes.
- ❖ Serve once; mixture is completely frozen and appears as crushed ice after about 3 hours.

242) Honey bread pudding

Preparation Time: 15-20 minutes　　　**Cooking Time**: 40-45 minutes　　　**Servings: 4**

Ingredients:

- ✓ 6 cups of white bread cubes
- ✓ 1 teaspoon of pure vanilla extract
- ✓ ¼ cup of honey

Directions:

- ❖ Lightly oil a buttered 8-by-8-inch baking dish; set aside.
- ❖ Whisk together the rice milk, eggs, egg whites, sugar and vanilla in a medium bowl.
- ❖ Add the bread cubes and stir until covered with the bread.

Ingredients:

- ✓ 2 large egg whites
- ✓ 2 eggs
- ✓ 1½ cups plain rice milk
- ❖ Move the mixture and cover with plastic wrap in the baking dish.
- ❖ Keep the dish in the refrigerator for a minimum of 3 hours.
- ❖ Preheat the oven to 325°F.
- ❖ Remove the plastic wrap from the pan and bake the pudding for 35-40 minutes, or until a knife inserted in the middle comes out clean and golden brown.
- ❖ Serve hot.

243) Vanilla Couscous Pudding

Preparation Time: 15-20 minutes　　　**Cooking Time**: 20 minutes　　　**Servings: 4**

Ingredients:

- ✓ 1 cup of couscous
- ✓ ¼ teaspoon ground cinnamon
- ✓ ½ cup of honey

Directions:

- ❖ In a large saucepan, combine the water, rice milk and vanilla seeds over medium-low heat.
- ❖ Bring the milk to a gentle boil, reduce the heat to low and let the milk simmer for about 10 minutes to allow the vanilla flavor to enter the milk.
- ❖ Remove the saucepan from the heat.

Ingredients:

- ✓ 1 vanilla pod, separated
- ✓ ½ cup of water
- ✓ 1½ cups plain rice milk
- ❖ Pull out the vanilla pod and remove the seeds from the pod into the hot milk with the tip of a sharp knife.
- ❖ Stir in the cinnamon and sugar.
- ❖ Cover the dish, stir the couscous and let it sit for about 10 minutes.
- ❖ Using a fork, fluff the couscous before eating.

244)   Raspberry Brule

Preparation Time: 15-20 minutes   **Cooking Time**: 1 minutes   **Servings: 4**

Ingredients:

- ✓ 1 cup fresh raspberries
- ✓ ¼ teaspoon ground cinnamon
- ✓ ¼ cup of brown sugar, divided

Directions:

- ❖ Preheat the baking oven.
- ❖ Beat the heavy cream, cream cheese, 2 teaspoons brown sugar and cinnamon together in a small bowl for about 4 minutes or until very smooth and fluffy.
- ❖ Divide raspberries evenly among four ramekins (4 ounces).

Ingredients:

- ✓ ½ cup plain cream cheese, room temperature
- ✓ ½ cup light sour cream

- ❖ Spoon the cream cheese combination over the berries and smooth the tops.
- ❖ Store ramekins until ready to eat dessert in the refrigerator, sealed.
- ❖ On each ramekin, sprinkle 1/2 tablespoon brown sugar evenly.
- ❖ Place the ramekins on a baking sheet until the sugar is caramelized and golden brown, and bake them 4 inches from the heating element.
- ❖ Remove from microwave. Let them rest for 1 minute and serve rules

245)   Victoria Sponge Cake

Preparation Time: 10 minutes   **Cooking Time**: 35 minutes   **Servings: 4**

Ingredients:

- ✓ 50ml heavy cream
- ✓ A splash of milk (if necessary)
- ✓ 250g (9oz) of self-raising flour
- ✓ 4 medium eggs

Directions:

- ❖ Grease two shallow 8-inch cake pans and then line them with baking paper for baking. Preheat the oven to 180°C (160° F) / 350°s F / Gas 4.
- ❖ In a large bowl, include the melted butter and sugar and whisk until very pale and fluffy. This is likely to take about 5-10 minutes. This can be achieved in a standalone mixer, if needed.
- ❖ Apply one egg and one giant spoonful of flour to the mixture and beat again. Until all the eggs are included, repeat this process. Sift out excess flour and then use a large metal spoon to fold over the mixture.

Ingredients:

- ✓ 250g (9oz) caster sugar
- ✓ 250g (9oz) unsalted butter, well softened
- ✓ About 5 tablespoons of raspberry jam (add more or less for your favorite flavor)
- ❖ Add a splash of milk if the dough doesn't have a droopy consistency (i.e., it slides off a spoon quickly).
- ❖ Spread the mixture between the two pans, smooth the surface and bake for 25 minutes.
- ❖ They should sandwich together until the cakes have been boiled and cooled. Whip the heavy cream until soft peaks form. Spread the jelly on one of the cakes and then spread the whipped cream on top of the jam. Place on top of the second cake and sift in the powdered sugar for decoration.

PART III: INTRODUCTION TO THE BENEFITS OF THE RENAL DIET

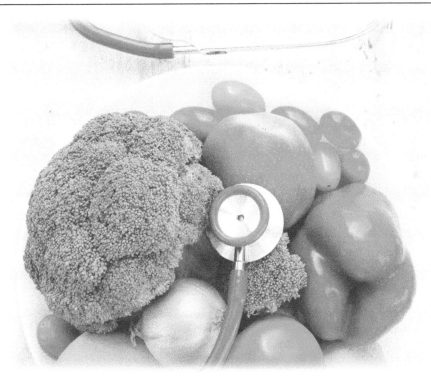

You need an eating plan that includes a kidney diet if you have a kidney disorder. It will help you stay healthy if you notice what you eat and drink. The facts in this section apply to individuals with kidney disease who are not treated with dialysis. Talk to your renal dietitian (an expert in diet and nutrition for patients with kidney disease) to see what meal pattern works best for you. Ask always your doctor to help you find a nutritionist. Private insurance and Medicare policies can help pay for dietary appointments. As part of dietary hygiene measures, nutritional counseling should be the first recommendation to the patient. Dietary care has always been considered important in chronic kidney disease (CKD), both as a renoprotective antiproteinuric measure in the predialysis phase and to prevent overweight and malnutrition at all stages, the latter in dialysis patients. The first premise is to ensure adequate caloric, protein, and mineral support. Never should insufficient nutrition be the price to pay for a supposedly adequate diet. Nutritional recommendations must be tailored to the ideal - not real - weight and adjusted for the patient's energy expenditure and physical activity. Why is it so important to follow a nutrition plan? The things we eat and drink can affect our health. People with diabetes can help control blood sugar levels by choosing what to eat and drink very carefully. Controlling blood pressure and diabetes can help prevent kidney disease from getting worse. A kidney diet helps prevent kidney damage. The kidney diet limits certain foods and prevents the minerals in those foods from building up in the body. Kidney diet basics With all meal plans, including the kidney diet, you must keep track of the number of specific nutrients you consume, such as: - Calories - Protein - Fat - Carbohydrates - Etc. All the information you need to keep track of your consumption is contained in a "nutritional information" label. Use the nutritional information section on meal labels to learn more about the foods you eat. Nutritional information will tell you how much protein, carbohydrates, fat, and sodium are in each serving of that meal. This can help you choose foods rich in the nutrients you need and low in the ones you should limit. Look at the nutrition facts, a few key areas will give you the information you need: calories you eat and drink are the source of your body's energy. Protein, carbohydrates, and dietary fat are the products of calories. Calorie needs to depend on your age, gender, body size, and activity level. You can adjust your calorie intake based on your weight. Some people limit their calories; others need to eat more calories Protein-Protein is one of the basic components of the body. To grow, heal and stay healthy, the body needs protein. Your skin, hair, and nails may be weakened by too little protein. But there is too much protein. To improve your health and mood, the amount of protein you eat may need to be adjusted. The number of protein you should consume depends on your body size, activity level, and health problems. This is because a high-protein diet can hinder kidney function and cause damage. Protein intake recommendations vary depending on the stage of the patient. In ACKD, moderate restriction of protein intake is recommended; in dialysis patients, intakes should be higher to compensate for the catabolic nature of the technique. Find out what foods are low and high in protein. Remember that just because a meal is low in protein doesn't mean you can consume it in high amounts. Low-protein meals High-protein meals Bread Red meat Fruits Chicken Vegetables Fish Pasta and rice Eggs Protein restriction in ACKD The kidney is the natural route of eliminating nitrogenous products. It is based on the fact that, unlike sugars and fats whose end product is H_2O and CO_2, the end product of protein metabolism is nitrogen, which is eliminated primarily by the kidneys in the form of urea. As renal failure progresses, these nitrogen products (along with phosphates, sulfates, and organic acids) accumulate in proportion to the loss of renal function. This gave rise to the principle of protein restriction and the kinetic model of urea for establishing dialysis dose. Protein restriction has been prevalent for decades (since 1918) and was the cornerstone of treatment when dialysis did not exist. Hydration ACKD is discussed at length elsewhere. For dialysis patients, it is recommended that they drink as much fluid as is eliminated with urine during this period, plus an additional 500-750cc. Regarding the patient's weight, the dialytic gain should not exceed 4-5% of his or her dry weight. In PD, fluid balance is continuous, but peritoneal ultrafiltration capacity is limited, so moderate fluid restriction and adjustment of peritoneal balances are recommended. Salt intake Limiting salt intake is a classic indication, both in patients with ACKD and renal replacement therapy. It is important to prevent salt retention, an adjuvant in blood pressure control, and even reduces proteinuria and facilitates the effect of renin-angiotensin axis blockers. We must consider it very important to verify saline intake to promote adherence to this prescription objectively. The most convenient method of monitoring salt intake is urinary sodium excretion, and we must emphasize the importance of measuring urinary sodium during routine visits. Now, is urinary sodium useful as an indicator of salt intake? The answer is not easy to find in the literature, and the information must be sought in classic books on human physiology. Under normal conditions, the fecal excretion of sodium is less than 0.5% of the intestinal content of the ion due to its rapid and efficient absorption by the intestinal mucosa. Therefore, if we consider that the intestine absorbs almost all of the ingested sodium, urinary sodium elimination is a good reflection of salt intake. Although there is always the risk of inadequate 24-hour urine collection, several studies have shown that it is the most practical method to check salt intake. Fat To stay healthy, you need some fat in your eating plan. Fat gives you energy and helps you eat certain vitamins. However, too much fat can lead to heart and weight gain. Limit fat in your diet and select healthier fats if possible. The healthiest fat or "good" fat is called unsaturated fat. Examples of unsaturated fats include: - Olive oil - Peanut oil - Corn oil. Unsaturated fats can help lower cholesterol levels. Try to eat unsaturated fats if you need to gain weight. Limit unsaturated fats in your eating plan if you need to lose weight.   Modesty is key, as always. There can be too many problems with "good" fats. Saturated fats, also called "bad" fats, can increase your risk of heart disease and cholesterol levels. Examples of saturated fats include: - Butter - Lard - Shortening - Meats. Limit these fats in your eating plan. Instead, choose healthy, unsaturated fats. Reducing the amount of fat in meat and removing the skin from chicken or turkey can also limit saturated fat. Trans fats should also be avoided, since this type of fat increases "bad" cholesterol. If this happens, heart disease is more likely to lead to kidney damage. Too much sodium can cause thirst, which can cause bloating and increase blood pressure. This can damage your kidneys and make it harder for your heart to work. One of the best ways to stay healthy is to limit your sodium intake. Control sodium in your eating plan: - Don't add salt to your food when you cook or eat. Try to cook with fresh herbs, lemon juice, or unsalted spices. - Choose fresh or frozen vegetables rather than canned vegetables. Eliminate from canned vegetable the liquid and rinse them to remove salt before cooking or eating them. - Avoid processed meats such as ham, bacon, hot dogs or chorizo, and luncheon meats. - Eat fresh fruits and vegetables instead of cookies or other salty snacks. - Avoid canned soups and frozen meals that are high in sodium. - Avoid foods such as olives and pickles that have been pickled. - Limit high-sodium condiments such as soy sauce, barbecue sauce, or ketchup. Important! Important. Pay attention to salt substitutes or "low sodium" foods. Work with your dietitian to find foods that are low in sodium and potassium. Portions It's a great start to choosing healthy foods, but overeating can be a problem. The other component of a healthy diet is portion control or watching how much you eat. To control portions: - On all foods, check the label for nutrition facts and learn the serving size. Most packages have more than one serving. With nutrition facts labels, fresh foods, such as fruits and vegetables, don't come. Ask your dietitian for a list of fresh foods for nutrition and advice on properly measuring portions. - Eat slowly, and when you are no longer hungry, stop eating. It takes your stomach about 20 minutes to tell your brain that it is already full. When you are doing something else, like watching TV or driving, avoid eating. You don't know how much you've eaten when you're distracted. - Don't eat directly from the food package. Instead, take a portion of food and put the bag or box at a distance. Controlling portion sizes is important for any eating plan. It is even more important on a kidney diet because you may need to limit how much you eat or drink. What is the difference between kidney diets?

When kidneys don't work well, waste and fluids build up in your body. These extra fluids and wastes can cause heart, bone, and other health problems over time. A kidney diet plan can limit the number of certain minerals and fluids you consume. This can keep you from accumulating and causing problems with the extra waste and fluids. Depending on your stage of kidney disease, it will depend on how strict you need to be with your plan. There may be little limit to what you eat or drink in the early stages of kidney disease. As time goes on and kidney disease worsens, your doctor may recommend limiting: - Potassium - The match - Liquids Potassium Potassium is a mineral found in almost all foods. Your body needs a certain level of potassium for your muscles to work, but too much potassium can be dangerous. Your potassium level can be very high or very low when your kidneys are not working well. Muscle cramps, problems with your heartbeat, and muscle weakness can be caused by too much or too little potassium. Limit the amount of potassium you eat if you have kidney disease. Ask your doctor or nutritionist if you should restrict your potassium intake. Find out which foods contain high and low levels of potassium. Your nutritionist can help you figure out how healthy it is to eat small amounts of your favorite high-potassium foods. Eat this (Low Potassium Foods) Instead of (High Potassium Foods) Apples, grapes, strawberries, pineapple, and plow, Avocado (avocado), bananas, melons, oranges, plums, and raisins. Cauliflower, onions, peppers, radishes, summer squash, and lettuce Artichokes, squash, bananas, spinach, potatoes, and tomatoes. Pita, tortillas and white bread, bran products, and granola. Beef, chicken and white rice, Beans, brown or wild rice (baked, black, pinto, etc.) Pair Phosphorus is found in almost all foods as a mineral. It maintains healthy bones by utilizing calcium and vitamin D. Healthy kidneys keep phosphorus in the body at the right level. Phosphorus can build up if your kidneys don't work well. In your blood, too much phosphorus can easily cause bones to break. There must be phosphorus limits for many people with kidney disease. Ask your doctor if phosphorus should be limited. Your doctor may prescribe a medicine called a phosphorus binder, depending on your stage of kidney disease. This may keep your blood from building up phosphorus. You may need to control the amount of phosphorus you eat in your diet. To get an idea of how to make healthy choices if you need to limit phosphorus in your diet, use the chart below Eat this (Low phosphorus meals) Instead of this (High phosphorus foods) Italian, French or sourdough bread. Whole grain bread. Corn or rice cereal and cream of wheat. Bran and oat cereals. Unsalted popcorn. Dried fruit and sunflower seeds. Light-colored soda or lemonade. Dark-colored sodas. Our bodies need survival water, but you may not need it as much if you have kidney disease. This is why they don't remove extra fluids as they should if your kidneys are damaged. Too much liquid can be dangerous for your body. High blood pressure, heart failure, and swelling can occur. The extra fluids that collect near your lungs can make it hard to breathe. Your doctor may ask you to limit the number of fluids you drink, depending on the stage of your kidney disease and your treatment. You will need to limit the amount you take if your doctor asks you to do so. Some foods that contain water will also need to be eliminated. Soups and foods that dissolve have a lot of water, such as cream of icing and jelly. Many fruits and vegetables also have high water content. To control how much you drink, you need to limit liquids, measure amounts of fluid and drink from small glasses. To prevent thirst, limit the amount of salt. Sometimes you may feel thirsty. You can do the following to help relieve thirst: - Chew gum. - Rinse your mouth. - Suck on an ice cube, mint, or hard candy (remember to choose a sugar-free candy if you have diabetes).

SPECIAL DIETARY CONCERNS

Vitamins

Following an eating plan with a kidney diet can prevent your body from getting enough of the vitamins and minerals you need. To help you get the correct levels of vitamins and minerals, your dietitian may suggest a supplement created for people with kidney disease.

Therapists or dietitians may also suggest a particular type of vitamin D, folic acid, or an iron pill help prevent some side effects typical of kidney diseases, such as bone disease and anemia. However, regular use of many vitamins may not be healthy for you if you have kidney disease. This is because they may contain a lot or too little vitamin.

AFTER DIABETIC MEAL FOR KIDNEYS

If you have diabetes, you need to check your blood sugar levels to avoid kidney damage. A doctor or nutritionist can help you create a meal plan that allows you to control your blood sugar levels while limiting sodium, phosphorus, potassium, and water. Diabetes educators can also learn how to control blood sugar levels. Ask your doctor to introduce you to a diabetes educator in your area. Private insurance and Medicare can help you pay for reservations with diabetes educators.

THE RENAL DIET

To decrease the amount of waste in the blood, individuals with impaired kidney function must adhere to a kidney diet. Waste in the blood is produced by liquids and foods that are ingested. Because kidney activity is impaired, the kidneys do not adequately filter or extract the waste. If the excess remains in the blood, it negatively affects the patient's electrolyte levels. Maintaining a renal diet can help improve kidney function and delay the progression of kidney failure.

A diet deficient in phosphorus, protein, and sodium is a renal diet. A renal diet often emphasizes the value of consuming high-quality protein and typically limits fluids. Calcium and potassium will also need to be modified for specific patients. An individual's body is different, so each patient needs to work with a renal dietitian to create a diet customized to the patient's needs.

Substances that are essential for screening to support a renal diet are listed below:

Sodium

What is the role of sodium in the body?

In particular natural foods, sodium is a mineral that is present. Most individuals think of sodium and salt as synonymous. However, salt is a complex of sodium and chloride. Therefore, the food we consume may include salt, which may contain other sources of sodium. Because of the added salt, refined foods also produce higher levels of sodium.

Sodium is one of the three main electrolytes in the body (chloride and potassium are the other two). Electrolytes regulate the fluids that enter and leave the body's tissues and cells. Sodium contributes to:

- Regulating nerve activity and muscle contraction
- Controlling blood volume and blood pressure
- Balancing the amount of fluid stored or eliminated from the body
- Regulating the acid-base balance of the blood

Why should renal patients monitor their sodium intake?

When fluid and sodium build up in the bloodstream and tissues, it can cause:

- Edema: swelling of the hands, face, and legs
- Increased thirst
- Shortness of breath: fluid builds up in the lungs, making it difficult to breathe.
- Heart failure: The heart will work too hard with the extra fluid in the bloodstream, making it weak and enlarged.
- High blood pressure

How can patients control their sodium intake?

- For portion sizes, be very careful.
- Always read the label on the food. Always list the sodium content.
- Choose fresh vegetables and fruits or frozen and canned products with no added salt.
- Use fresh meat instead of packaged meat.
- Compare brands and use those with the lowest sodium content.
- Avoid processed products.
- Prepare at home and do NOT add salt.
- Use spices that do not have "salt" in the title (prefer garlic powder instead of garlic salt).
- Limit total sodium level per meal to 400 mg and per snack to 150 mg.

Potassium

In maintaining a regular heartbeat and proper muscle function, potassium plays an important role. The kidneys help keep the correct amount of potassium in the body and remove excess amounts in the urine.

Why should patients with kidneys monitor their potassium intake?

High potassium in the blood is known as hyperkalemia which can trigger

- An abnormal heartbeat
- Weakness in the muscles
- Death
- Heart attacks
- Slow pulse

How can patients control their potassium intake?

In some foods, phosphorus can be identified. Therefore, to better control amounts of phosphorus, patients with impaired kidney function can consult a renal dietitian.

Tips to help keep phosphorus at healthy levels:

- For portion sizes, pay close attention to.
- Know which foods have less phosphorus.
- Eating fresh fruits and vegetables.
- Eat small amounts of protein-rich foods for snacks and meals.
- Avoid packaged foods that contain added phosphorus. On ingredient labels, look for phosphorus and words with "PHOS" in them.
- Ask your doctor about using phosphate binders with meals.
- Keep a food diary

Protein

Protein is usually absorbing waste products are produced that are purified by the nephrons of the kidneys. Then, the waste is turned into the urine with the help of other kidney proteins. But, on the other hand, damaged kidneys refuse to eliminate protein waste, and it accumulates in the blood.

For patients with chronic kidney disorders, adequate protein intake is derrick. The amount varies depending on the level of the disease. Protein is necessary for tissue maintenance and other bodily roles. Still, according to the renal dietitian or nephrologist, it is essential to consume the amount prescribed for the particular stage of the disease.

Fluids

For patients in the later stages of kidney disease, fluid management is essential because regular fluid intake can contribute to fluid build-up in the body that can become detrimental. People on dialysis also have a reduced flow of urine, so the additional fluid in the body will put undue pressure on the person's lungs and heart.

Based on urine output and dialysis conditions, a patient's fluid allocation is measured individually. Therefore, asking the nephrologist/nutritionist for fluid intake guidelines is essential.

To monitor fluid intake, patients should:

- Do not drink more than prescribed by the physician.
- Count all foods that dissolve at room temperature.
- Know the number of fluids used for cooking.

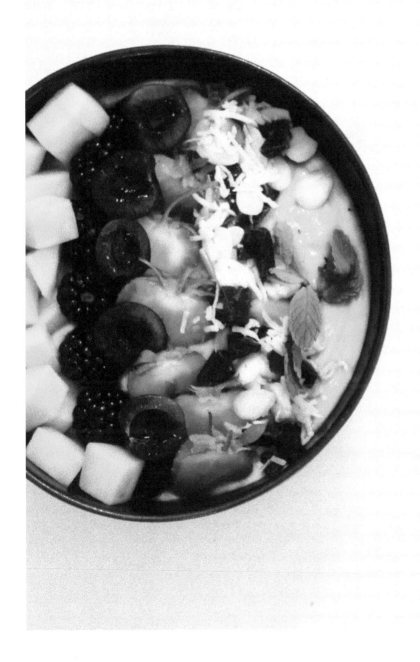

246) Cappuccino at home

Preparation Time: 10 min   **Cooking Time**: 10 min   **Servings: 2**

Ingredients:

- ✓ One cup of low-fat (1%) or fat-free milk

Directions:

- ❖ Heat milk over medium heat in a small saucepan until it steams. (Or heat in a microwave for about 1 minute on high heat).
- ❖ Meanwhile, bring fresh water to the base of the coffee maker up to the steam nozzle.
- ❖ To the basket, transfer the coffee beans by screwing it up to the top. Bring to a boil at high temperature and cook until the coffee has stopped splashing under the lid through the longitudinal spout.

Ingredients:

- ✓ Three tablespoons of ground coffee beans
- ❖ Remove that from the heat of the temperature.
- ❖ In a blender, pour in the hot milk and process once sticky.
- ❖ Divide the coffee into two coffee cups. Pour the same amount of milk from the blender to cover the coffee with the remaining milk, then pour in. Serve hot.

247) Green Tea Ginger

Preparation Time: 5 min   **Cooking Time**: 8 min   **Servings: 1**

Ingredients:

- ✓ Two quarter-sized strips of fresh, unpeeled ginger
- ✓ 3/4 cup of water

Directions:

- ❖ In a small skillet, place the ginger and beat the pieces with the edge of a wooden spoon.
- ❖ Include water and at high temperature, bring to a boil.

Ingredients:

- ✓ One green tea bag

- ❖ In a cup, insert a tea bag. With the ginger, pour in the hot water. Allow 2 to 3 minutes for steeping.
- ❖ Remove the ginger and tea bag, using only a spoon.
- ❖ Drink warm.

248) Buckwheat crepes

Preparation Time: 5 min   **Cooking Time**: 10 min   **Servings: 6**

Ingredients:

- ✓ One cup of buckwheat flour
- ✓ 1/3 cup whole wheat flour
- ✓ One beaten egg

Directions:

- ❖ Mix and match all the elements in the mixing bowl and beat until you have a consistent batter.
- ❖ Heat nonstick skillet for three minutes on high heat.
- ❖ Ladle in a small amount of batter. And straighten the pan in the style of a crepe.

Ingredients:

- ✓ One cup of skimmed milk
- ✓ One teaspoon of olive oil
- ✓ 1/2 teaspoon ground cinnamon
- ❖ For 1 min, cook it and flip it to the other side. Cook it for an extra 30 seconds.
- ❖ With the leftover batter, repeat the previous procedure.

249) Muffins with carrots

Preparation Time: 5 min   **Cooking Time**: 10 min   **Servings: 5**

Ingredients:

- ✓ 1 1/2 cups whole wheat flour
- ✓ 1/2 cup stevia

Ingredients:

- ✓ 1 single egg
- ✓ Fresh Blueberries 1 cup

- ✓ 1 tablespoon baking powder
- ✓ 1/2 teaspoon cinnamon powder
- ✓ 1/2 tablespoon of cooking soda
- ✓ 1/4 cup of natural apple juice
- ✓ Olive oil about 1/4 cup

Directions:

- ❖ Combine the flour and stevia in a large bowl, baking powder, baking soda and cinnamon and mix well.
- ❖ Include apple juice, oil, blueberries, carrots, cranberries, ginger and pecans. But very well shaken.

- ✓ Two carrots, grated
- ✓ Ginger 2 tablespoons, brushed
- ✓ 1/4 cup chopped pecans
- ✓ Cooking spray

- ❖ Grease a muffin pan with cooking spray, divide the muffin mixture, place in the oven and bake for thirty minutes at 375 degrees Fahrenheit
- ❖ Divide muffins between plates and serve for breakfast. Love!

250) Chia seed breakfast mix

Preparation Time: 8 hours   **Cooking Time**: none   **Servings: 4**

Ingredients:

- ✓ Old fashioned oats with 2 cups
- ✓ Four tablespoons of chia seeds
- ✓ Four tablespoons of coconut sugar

Directions:

- ❖ Integrate oats with chia seeds, sugar, milk, lemon and chia seeds in a cup.

Ingredients:

- ✓ THREE cups of coconut milk
- ✓ 1 teaspoon of lemon zest, minced
- ✓ Blueberries 1 cup
- ❖ Stir in zest and blueberries, divide into cups and keep in refrigerator. For 8 hours.
- ❖ For breakfast, serve. Enjoy!

251) High Energy Porridge

Preparation Time: 15-20 min   **Cooking Time**: 15 min   **Servings: 4**

Ingredients:

- ✓ 200ml whole milk
- ✓ 35g (1¼oz) porridge oats

Directions:

- ❖ In a skillet, combine all ingredients, heat the pan and boil the mixture for about 3-4 minutes.

Ingredients:

- ✓ Optional: add a little cream and syrup or jam for extra energy
- ❖ Or you can cook it for about 1-2 minutes in the microwave, stirring at 30 second intervals.

252) Blueberry and Pineapple Smoothie

Preparation Time: 15 min   **Cooking Time**: None   **Servings: 2**

Ingredients:

- ✓ ½ cup of water
- ✓ ½ apple
- ✓ ½ cup of English cucumber

Directions:

- ❖ In a blender, add the blueberries, cucumber, pineapple, apple and water and combine until thick.

Ingredients:

- ✓ ½ cup of pineapple chunks
- ✓ 1 cup of frozen blueberries

- ❖ Pour smoothie into 2 glasses and enjoy.

253)   The Beach Boy Omelette

Preparation Time: 5 min   **Cooking Time**: 5-10 min   **Servings**: 1

Ingredients:

- ✓   2 sprigs of parsley
- ✓   1 tablespoon of soy milk
- ✓   2 egg whites
- ✓   1 whole egg

Directions:

- ❖   Heat the oil and add the onion and pepper. Sauté for about 2 minutes.
- ❖   Add the browns with the shredded hash and simmer for another 5 minutes.
- ❖   Whip the milk and eggs and place the mixture in a separate omelet tray.

Ingredients:

- ✓   2 tablespoons of frozen shredded hash browns
- ✓   2 tablespoons of diced green bell pepper
- ✓   2 tablespoons of diced onion
- ✓   1 tablespoon of canola oil
- ❖   Cook until your omelet is firm.
- ❖   Place the hash brown mixture in the center of the omelet and roll the omelet up.
- ❖   Garnish with new parsley to serve.

254)   Chocolate and Peanut Butter Smoothie

Preparation Time: 5 min   **Cooking Time**: 10 min   **Servings**: 2

Ingredients:

- ✓   A ripe banana, at least overnight, stored
- ✓   2/3 cup low-fat milk (1%)
- ✓   2/3 cup low-fat yogurt
- ✓   Crispy peanut butter 2 tablespoons.

Directions:

- ❖   Slice and chop the banana into pieces.
- ❖   Blend bananas in a blender with milk, yogurt, peanut butter, sugar substitute (if using), cocoa powder and ice cubes.

Ingredients:

- ✓   Two teaspoons of unsweetened cocoa powder
- ✓   One tablespoon of amber agave nectar (optional)
- ✓   Four ice cubes

- ❖   Load into two large glasses and serve immediately.

255)   Cabbage and apple smoothie

Preparation Time: 8 min   **Cooking Time**: 10 min   **Servings**: 1

Ingredients:

- ✓   1 cup kale leaves, well washed, shredded and loose
- ✓   1/2 cup Jonathan or Gala sweet fruit, cored and coarsely chopped
- ✓   1/3 cup apple cider vinegar

Directions:

- ❖   In a blender, blend all ingredients until creamy.

Ingredients:

- ✓   2 tablespoons of sunflower seeds
- ✓   Six ice cubes
- ✓   Eight leaves of healthy mint

- ❖   Sprinkle into a tall glass and serve instantly.

256) Lassi mango

Preparation Time: 15 min   **Cooking Time**: none   **Servings: 1**

Ingredients:
- ✓ One ripe mango, pitted, sliced and coarsely chopped 1/2 cup
- ✓ Smooth without fat
- ✓ yogurt

Directions:
- ❖ Blend the mango cubes, yogurt, milk and ice until smooth.

Ingredients:
- ✓ 1/2 cup fat-free milk
- ✓ Three ice cubes
- ✓ Pinch of ground cardamom (optional)

- ❖ Pour into a long glass. Sprinkle with cardamom, if using. Serve immediately.

257) Papaya and Coconut Breakfast Smoothie

Preparation Time: 11 min   **Cooking Time**: none   **Servings: 2**

Ingredients:
- ✓ One ripe papaya, seed and skin removed and cut into 1-inch chunks
- ✓ A cup of low-fat yogurt
- ✓ One cup of water with coconut (not coconut milk)

Directions:
- ❖ In a processor, puree all materials, such as sweetener (if used).

Ingredients:
- ✓ Two tablespoons of wheat germ
- ✓ 1/2 teaspoon of zero-calorie sweetener (optional)

- ❖ Pour into 2 large glasses and serve.

258) Whole wheat strawberry and maple compote pancakes

Preparation Time: 3 min   **Cooking Time**: 6 min   **Servings: 6**

Ingredients:
- ✓ Compote
- ✓ Fresh strawberries, one pound (1 quart) cored and finely chopped 1/4 cup maple syrup
- ✓ Pancakes
- ✓ One cup of whole wheat pasta flour
- ✓ 1/2 cup superfine whole wheat flour
- ✓ Sugar per 1 teaspoon.

Directions:
- ❖ Compote: In a medium bowl, combine the strawberries and maple syrup.
- ❖ Leave the strawberries at room temperature to allow the fluids to be released at room temperature. A minimum of 1 hour and up to 4 hours.
- ❖ To make the pancakes: preheat the oven to 200°F. In a medium bowl, mix together the whole wheat dough flour, unbleached flour, sugar, salt and baking powder.
- ❖ Mix the milk, egg and egg whites and the 2 tablespoons of oil. Add the dry ingredients and mix until just combined.

Ingredients:
- ✓ 11/2 teaspoon baking powder
- ✓ 1/4 teaspoon. kosher salt.
- ✓ 11/2 cup low-fat milk (1%)
- ✓ 1 huge egg plus 2 big white eggs
- ✓ In a pump sprayer, two teaspoons of canola or corn oil, and more

- ❖ Over medium-high heat, heat a grill pan (ideally nonstick). Drizzle it with a little oil.
- ❖ For each pancake, add 1/4 cup of batter to grill pan. Cook until the top is done.
- ❖ The top of each pancake is covered with a bubble for about two minutes. Flip the pancakes over with a large spatula and bake for a few minutes until the undersides are golden brown, about 1 minute longer.
- ❖ On a baking sheet, move pancakes and keep leftover pancakes warm in the oven before preparing.

259) Blueberries and yogurt cornmeal waffles

Preparation Time: 5 min   **Cooking Time**: 10 min   **Servings**: 8

Ingredients:
- ✓ One cup unbleached whole wheat flour
- ✓ One cup of cornmeal that is really yellow
- ✓ Sugar 2 teaspoons
- ✓ 1½ teaspoon baking powder
- ✓ 1/4 teaspoon of kosher salt
- ✓ 1¾ cups low-fat milk (1%)

Ingredients:
- ✓ 1 tablespoon unsalted butter, melted
- ✓ 1 tablespoon canola or corn oil, plus more in a pump sprayer,
- ✓ Two main egg whites
- ✓ Two cups regular low-fat yogurt to serve, at room temperature,
- ✓ Two containers of blueberries (6 ounces) (about 2⅔ cups), at room temperature, to serve.
- ❖ In the batter, bring in the whites. Spray oil onto waffle iron. (Do not use nonstick spray with aerosol.) (Do not use nonstick spray with aerosol.) Pour 1 cup of batter into waffle iron (exact amount depends on scale of waffle iron) cover iron and cook according to manufacturer's instructions before is waffle golden brown.
- ❖ From the iron, cut out the waffle, move to a baking sheet and keep the oven warm when making the remaining waffles.
- ❖ Divide the squares into waffles. Stack 2 waffle squares on a plate for each serving.
- ❖ Top with 1/4 cup yogurt and 1/3 cup blueberries and serve immediately.

Directions:
- ❖ Preheat oven to 200°F. Preheat a nonstick waffle iron as per instructions from the maker.
- ❖ in a large bowl, mix together all the flour, cornmeal, sugar, baking powder and salt.
- ❖ Mix milk, melted butter and 1 tablespoon oil in a small bowl Add dry ingredients and stir with a wooden spoon until products are dry.
- ❖ Just lightly mixed with flour strips; should not over mix.
- ❖ Pull egg whites with an electric immersion blender into a separate bowl at high speed just until stiff peaks are reached and not dry.

260) Banana smoothie berries

Preparation Time: 5 min   **Cooking Time**: 10 min   **Servings**:

Ingredients:
- ✓ 1/2 ripe banana, ideally frozen
- ✓ 1/2 cup fresh or frozen blueberries
- ✓ 1/2 cup low-fat milk (1/%)

Directions:
- ❖ Slice and chop the banana into pieces.

Ingredients:
- ✓ 1/2 cup low-fat yogurt
- ✓ 1/4 teaspoon of vanilla extract
- ✓ 1 tablespoon of amber agave nectar (optional)
- ❖ Blend all products, such as sweetener (if used), when creamy, in a processor.
- ❖ Place in a tall glass and serve immediately.

261)   Tartlets with strawberries and cream cheese 1

Preparation Time: 5 min   **Cooking Time**: 10 min   **Servings: 1**

Ingredients:
- ✓ A slice of wholemeal bread
- ✓ Two tablespoons of fat-free spreadable cheese

Directions:
- ❖ In a toaster oven, toast the bread.

Ingredients:
- ✓ Two large strawberries cut into pieces
- ✓ Honey for 1 teaspoon (optional)
- ❖ Layer with the cream cheese and finish with the cream cheese on top of the strawberries.

262)   Broccoli and Pepper Jack Omelette

Preparation Time: 5 min   **Cooking Time**: 10 min   **Servings: 1**

Ingredients:
- ✓ In a pump sprayer, olive oil
- ✓ 1/2 cup of seasoned egg substitute liquid

Directions:
- ❖ Drizzle a small nonstick skillet over medium heat with oil and heat. Add the eggs, then
- ❖ Reposition and bake for about 15 seconds before the edges are set. Use a heat-resistant spatula
- ❖ Lift the edges of the egg substitute so that the uncooked liquid flows underneath.

Ingredients:
- ✓ A low-fat pepper jack cheese (2% milk) cut, torn into a few 1/4 cup pieces
- ✓ Broccoli (thawed frozen ones are fine), fried and sliced, reheated in the microwave,
- ❖ Continue to cook, lifting the sides every 15 seconds or so, until the omelet is done, about 1 1/2 minutes total.
- ❖ Remove from heat. Spread the rest of the cheese and broccoli omelet on top. Turn the pan marginally and use the spatula to fold the omelet again and again and into thirds. (From the heat of the omelet, the cheese will melt).
- ❖ Slide out. Place on a tray and then serve.

263)   Granola your way

Preparation Time: 5 min   **Cooking Time**: 7 min   **Servings: 10**

Ingredients:
- ✓ 1/4 cup medium brown sugar, rolled
- ✓ Two tablespoons of water
- ✓ One tablespoon of oil for the vegetables
- ✓ One teaspoon of cinnamon powder
- ✓ One tablespoon of maple extract or vanilla flavoring
- ✓ Four cups old-fashioned oats (rolled)

Directions:
- ❖ Mix brown sugar, water, oil, cinnamon and maple in a large dish.
- ❖ Flavor until sugar is dissolved. Insert oats and whisk in once lightly covered. On a large cookie sheet, spread evenly.
- ❖ Bake, stirring regularly and pushing the toasted sides into the center of the Granola, for about 40 minutes, until the oats are evenly crisp.

Ingredients:
- ✓ One cup of medium grapes
- ✓ 1/2 cup chopped dates
- ✓ 1/2 cup milk, fat-free, to serve
- ✓ Preheat the oven to 300°F.

- ❖ Remove from oven and stir in dates and raisins. Allow to cool completely.
- ❖ Store in an airtight place Up to 2 weeks in a jar.
- ❖ Place 1/2 cup of granola in a container for each serving and apply milk.

264) Muffins with spinach

Preparation Time: 10 min   **Cooking Time**: none   **Servings: 6**

Ingredients:

- ✓ Six eggs
- ✓ 1/2 cup fat-free milk
- ✓ 1 cup of low-fat crumbled cheese
- ✓ Spinach 4 ounces

Directions:

- ❖ Integrate eggs with milk, cheese, spinach and red spinach in a dish. Mix well with pepper and ham.

Ingredients:

- ✓ 1/2 cup of roasted red bell pepper, chopped
- ✓ Ham Two ounces, sliced
- ✓ Spray firing

- ❖ Oil a muffin pan with cooking spray, divide muffin mix, place in oven and bake for thirty minutes at 350 degrees Fahrenheit
- ❖ Divide the plates and serve them for breakfast. Enjoy!

265) Bowl of blueberry smoothie

Preparation Time: 15-20 min   **Cooking Time**: 15 min   **Servings: 1**

Ingredients:

- ✓ 2 tablespoons of shredded coconut
- ✓ 1 tablespoon of fiber cereal
- ✓ 2 strawberries
- ✓ 5 raspberries

Directions:

- ❖ In a blender, mix the blueberries
- ❖ Add the yogurt, milk and protein powder and mix until smooth.

Ingredients:

- ✓ 1/3 cup unsweetened vanilla almond milk
- ✓ ¼ cup of fat-free Greek yogurt
- ✓ 2 tablespoons of whey protein powder
- ✓ 1 cup blueberries, frozen
- ❖ Place the mixture in a bowl and top it off with some chopped raspberries, strawberries, cereal and coconut.

266) Egg white omelette with vegetables

Preparation Time: 10 min   **Cooking Time**: 10 min   **Servings: 2**

Ingredients:

- ✓ Six white eggs
- ✓ One tablespoon of water
- ✓ Two tablespoons of olive oil
- ✓ 1/2 yellow onion, sliced

Directions:

- ❖ In a medium bowl, beat egg whites, insert 1 tablespoon water and stir. With a fork until well blended.
- ❖ Heat 1 teaspoon oil in a medium-sized skillet over medium-high heat. Add the onions, tomatoes, asparagus and mushrooms and sauté until the vegetables are tender about 3-4 minutes. Remove from the skillet and dismiss.
- ❖ Introduce another teaspoon of oil into the skillet and allow it to heat for a minute or two. Bring the beaten eggs into the pan, swirling the pan as required so that the eggs cover the entire pan.

Ingredients:

- ✓ 1 sliced tomato
- ✓ 2-3 asparagus stalks, cut into small pieces
- ✓ 3-4 cut mushrooms

- ❖ Let the eggs settle along the edges of the pan, it will only take a few moments if the pan is hot enough. Using a spatula, slide the eggs away from the edges of the pan and turn the pan to allow the egg mixture to circulate over the surface of the pan. Repeat until the eggs are almost done but still soft in the center.
- ❖ Introduce the vegetable mixture into the center of the omelet. Fold one side of the omelet over the toppings. Slide onto a plate. Voila, it's safe to serve.

267) Breakfast salad with fruit and yogurt

Preparation Time: 10 min   **Cooking Time**: 15-20 min   **Servings: 6**

Ingredients:

- ✓ 2 cups of water
- ✓ 1/4 teaspoon salt
- ✓ 3/4 cup of quick-cooking brown rice
- ✓ 3/4 cup bulgur
- ✓ One large apple, peeled and diced

Directions:

- ❖ Heat water over high heat in a large pot until it boils.
- ❖ Integrate the salt, rice and bulgur into the mixture. Reduce heat, cover and simmer for ten minutes. Remove from heat and encourage to sit for 2 minutes, covered.

Ingredients:

- ✓ One large pear, peeled and chopped
- ✓ One orange, peeled and cut into pieces
- ✓ 1 cup dried cranberries
- ✓ 1 box (8 ounces) of low-fat or fat-free plain Greek yogurt
- ❖ Place the grains in a large bowl and chill in the refrigerator until chilled.
- ❖ Take cold grains out of the freezer. Add strawberries, pears, bananas Cranberries that are dry. Fold and gently whisk in yogurt until grains and fruit are set. Wrap completely.
- ❖ In bowls, serve.

268) Spiced pumpkin fritters

Preparation Time: 5 min   **Cooking Time**: 10 min   **Servings: 10**

Ingredients:

- ✓ Two cups of total wheat flour
- ✓ Two teaspoons of flour for cooking
- ✓ One teaspoon of cooking soda
- ✓ One teaspoon of cinnamon
- ✓ 1/2 teaspoon of nutmeg
- ✓ 1/2 teaspoon ground ginger

Directions:

- ❖ Mix flour, baking powder, baking powder and baking soda together in a mixing bowl. 2. Nutmeg, cinnamon and ginger.
- ❖ Mix brown sugar, egg yolk and pumpkin in another dish. Stir in the milk.
- ❖ Pour the milk mixture with the dry ingredients into a pan. Stir until just melted. Do not over stir.

Ingredients:

- ✓ 1/4 cup brown sugar
- ✓ 1 egg yolk
- ✓ One cup of canned pumpkin
- ✓ Two tablespoons of coconut oil
- ✓ Skimmed milk Two cups
- ✓ Two egg whites
- ❖ In a skillet, beat egg whites until smooth. Fold the egg whites into the pancake batter.
- ❖ Over moderate heat, heat a nonstick skillet or large frying pan. Sprinkle with nonstick cooking.
- ❖ When the griddle is heated, 1/4 cup of ladle batter is applied to the pan. Cook for a while before the batter begins to bubble, flip, and cook until gently browned.

269) Lemon and zucchini muffins

Preparation Time: 5 min   **Cooking Time**: 10 min   **Servings**: 12

Ingredients:

- ✓ All-purpose flour - 2 cups
- ✓ 1/2 of a cup of sugar
- ✓ 1 tablespoon of flour for cooking
- ✓ 1/4 teaspoon salt
- ✓ 1/4 teaspoon of cinnamon
- ✓ 1/4 cup nutmeg

Directions:

- ❖ Preheat oven to 400°F. By gently spraying, ready the muffin tray or cooking spray or muffin liner.
- ❖ Integrate the flour, sugar, baking powder, salt, cinnamon, etc. into a blender bowl with the nutmeg.

Ingredients:

- ✓ 1 cup shredded zucchini
- ✓ 3/4 cup of fat-free milk
- ✓ Olive oil, 2 teaspoons
- ✓ Lemon juice for 2 tablespoons
- ✓ egg
- ✓ Non-stick mist for cooking
- ❖ Integrate the zucchini, milk, oil, lemon juice and egg into another dish. Mix well.
- ❖ Apply the zucchini solution to the flour combination. Stir before they are all mixed. Do not over mix.
- ❖ On the packaged muffin cups, add the batter. Bake for 20 minutes or until lightly browned.

270) English Muffin Breakfast

Preparation Time: 5 min   **Cooking Time**: 8 min   **Servings**: 1

Ingredients:

- ✓ 1⁄2 whole wheat English muffin
- ✓ One piece of low-fat Swiss cheese (2% milk), cut into pieces to fit the muffin Olive oil in a sprayer with pumps

Directions:

- ❖ Toast the English muffin in a grill or microwave toaster. Turn off the toaster
- ❖ Cover muffin with cheese slices and let stand until cheese begins to melt from heat generated for about 30 seconds. Move to a plate.
- ❖ Meanwhile, brush oil into a small nonstick skillet and cook over medium heat.
- ❖ Apply the egg substitute and bake for about 15 seconds before securing the edges.

Ingredients:

- ✓ 1⁄2 cup of seasoned egg substitute liquid
- ✓ 11⁄2 teaspoons coarsely diced shallots (green part only)
- ❖ Using a heat-resistant spatula, lift the sides of the egg substitute so that the uncooked liquid underneath flows out. Continue to cook, lifting the sides about every 15 seconds before the egg combination is done, for a total of 11⁄2 minutes. Using the spatula,
- ❖ To produce a sturdy "patty," fold the sides of the beaten egg into the core about 2 inches wide.

271) Apple Pancake Rings

Preparation Time: 5 min   **Cooking Time**: 1-2 min   **Servings: 20**

Ingredients:

- ✓ ½ teaspoon of cinnamon
- ✓ ¾ cup of frying oil
- ✓ 1 tablespoon of canola oil
- ✓ 1/3 cup of almond milk
- ✓ 1/3 cup low fat milk 1%

Directions:

- ❖ Peel and core the apples. From each apple, cut 5 circles, 1/2" thick.
- ❖ Sift together the rice, baking powder and two teaspoons of sugar.
- ❖ In a separate dish, combine the egg, almond yogurt, milk and 1 tablespoon oil.
- ❖ Combine the egg and dry mixtures before they are combined.
- ❖ In a deep skillet, boil 1 inch of cooking oil.

Ingredients:

- ✓ 1 beaten egg
- ✓ 1 teaspoon baking powder
- ✓ 6 tablespoons of sugar
- ✓ 1 cup white flour
- ✓ 4 large cooking apples
- ❖ Dip the apple rings in the batter and fry until golden brown or 1 to 1/2 minute.
- ❖ Drain them on cloth towels.
- ❖ Combine remaining sugar with cinnamon and sprinkle over patties.

272) Apple Oatmeal with Cinnamon

Preparation Time: 7 min   **Cooking Time**: 10 min   **Servings: 8**

Ingredients:

- ✓ 2 cups steel cut oats
- ✓ Water Eight cups
- ✓ Cinnamon - 1 teaspoon.
- ✓ 1/2 teaspoon of allspice
- ✓ Nutmeg 1/2 teaspoon.

Directions:

- ❖ Spray non-stick spray on a slow stove.
- ❖ Place all the items in the pot over low heat except for the nuts. Stir enough to make a paste.

Ingredients:

- ✓ 1/4 cup brown sugar
- ✓ 1 teaspoon of vanilla extraction
- ✓ Two apples, sliced
- ✓ 1 cup of raisins
- ✓ 1/2 cup unsalted, fried, diced walnuts
- ❖ Set the pot to low and cook for eight hours.
- ❖ Offer with diced walnuts.

273) Hot mixed cereals

Preparation Time: 10 min   **Cooking Time**: 25 min   **Servings: 4**

Ingredients:

- ✓ ½ teaspoon ground cinnamon
- ✓ 6 tablespoons of plain uncooked couscous
- ✓ 1 cup peeled and sliced apple
- ✓ 2 tablespoons whole uncooked buckwheat

Directions:

- ❖ Heat the water and milk in a medium saucepan over medium-high heat.
- ❖ Bring the bulgur, buckwheat and apple to a boil.
- ❖ Lower the heat and simmer, stirring regularly, for 20-25 minutes or until the bulgur is soft.

Ingredients:

- ✓ 6 tablespoons of uncooked bulgur
- ✓ 1¼ cup of vanilla rice milk
- ✓ 2¼ cups of water

- ❖ Stir in the couscous and cinnamon and remove the casserole from the sun.
- ❖ For 10 minutes, let the pot sit, sealed, and then fluff the cereal with a fork before eating

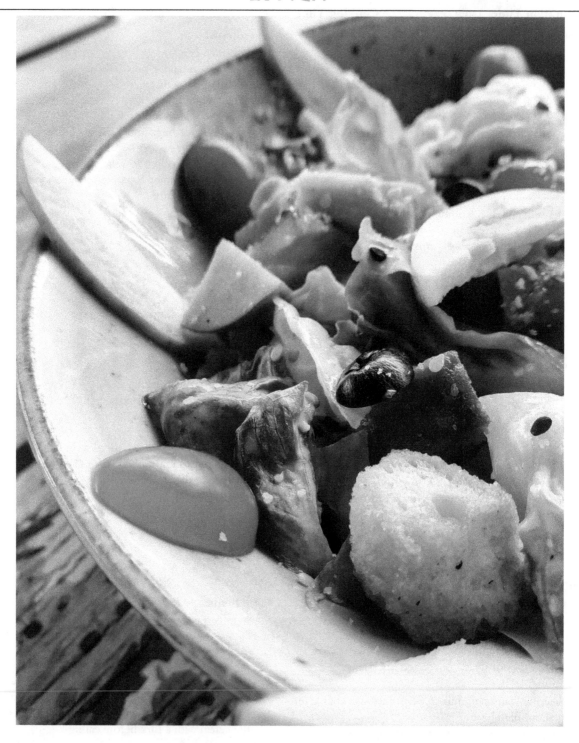

274)   Salmon with basil and garlic

Preparation Time: 10 minutes   **Cooking Time**: 4 minutes   **Servings: 2**

Ingredients:
- ✓ 2 tablespoons of avocado oil
- ✓ 4 salmon fillets, skinless

Directions:
- ❖ Heat the olive oil in a saucepan, add the fish and cook for 4 minutes.

Ingredients:
- ✓ 1 teaspoon of dried basil
- ✓ ½ teaspoon of garlic powder
- ❖ Sprinkle fried salmon with garlic powder and basil.

275)   Arctic char with mustard

Preparation Time: 10 minutes   **Cooking Time**: 10 minutes   **Servings: 2**

Ingredients:
- ✓ 1 tablespoon of mustard
- ✓ 1 tablespoon of olive oil

Directions:
- ❖ Sprinkle in the rosemary, olive oil and mustard.

Ingredients:
- ✓ ¼ teaspoon of dried rosemary
- ✓ 2 fillets of Arctic char
- ❖ Move the fish fillets to the baking sheet and bake for 10 minutes at 400F.

276)   Cod in yogurt sauce

Preparation Time: 10 minutes   **Cooking Time**: 12 minutes   **Servings: 2**

Ingredients:
- ✓ 1 teaspoon of sesame oil
- ✓ 4 cod fillets, boned and skinned
- ✓ ½ onion, diced

Directions:
- ❖ Rub cod fillets with dried cilantro, minced garlic and sesame oil.

Ingredients:
- ✓ ½ cup low-fat yogurt
- ✓ 1 tablespoon of dried coriander
- ✓ ½ teaspoon of minced garlic
- ❖ Place the fish in the skillet and cook for 3 minutes per side.
- ❖ Add the onion and fat yogurt. Cook the meat for an additional 12 minutes.

277)   Trout with parsley

Preparation Time: 10 minutes   **Cooking Time**: 8 minutes   **Servings: 2**

Ingredients:
- ✓ 1 tablespoon of dried parsley
- ✓ 6 trout fillets

Directions:
- ❖ Rub the trout fillets with the parsley.

Ingredients:
- ✓ 2 tablespoons margarine

- ❖ Then throw the margarine into the pan and let it melt.
- ❖ Add the fish fillets and cook for 4 minutes per side.

278) Paprika tuna steaks

Preparation Time: 10 minutes   **Cooking Time**: 2 minutes   **Servings: 4**

Ingredients:
- ✓ 1 teaspoon of avocado oil
- ✓ 4 tuna steaks, boneless

Ingredients:
- ✓ 1 teaspoon ground paprika

Directions:
- ❖ Rub fish with paprika and drizzle with avocado oil.
- ❖ Then transfer the tuna steaks to the preheated 400F grill and cook for 2 minutes per side.

279) Grilled Tilapia

Preparation Time: 10 minutes   **Cooking Time**: 3 minutes   **Servings: 2**

Ingredients:
- ✓ 1 tablespoon of sesame oil
- ✓ ½ teaspoon of ground black pepper

Ingredients:
- ✓ ½ teaspoon of garlic powder
- ✓ 4 medium fillets of tilapia
- ❖ Grill for 3 minutes per side in the preheated grill at 400F.

Directions:
- ❖ Sprinkle fish with garlic powder, ground black pepper and sesame oil.

280) Cod in orange juice

Preparation Time: 10 minutes   **Cooking Time**: 10 minutes   **Servings: 2**

Ingredients:
- ✓ 4 cod fillets, boneless
- ✓ 1 cup of orange juice
- ✓ 1 tablespoon chives, chopped

Ingredients:
- ✓ 1 tablespoon of olive oil
- ✓ ½ teaspoon of white pepper

- ❖ Add the chives and orange juice.
- ❖ For 10 minutes, cook the cod.

Directions:
- ❖ At medium pressure, pressure a skillet with oil.
- ❖ Sprinkle the fish with the white pepper and place in the hot oil.

281) Halibut fillets with tomato sauce

Preparation Time: 10 minutes   **Cooking Time**: 5 minutes   **Servings: 2**

Ingredients:
- ✓ 2 teaspoons of sesame oil
- ✓ 4 halibut fillets, skinless

Ingredients:
- ✓ 1 cup cherry tomatoes, halved
- ✓ 1 teaspoon of dried basil

- ❖ Sesame oil and cherry tomatoes are added.
- ❖ For 4 minutes, roast the flour and then stir well and simmer for another 5 minutes.

Directions:
- ❖ Sprinkle the basil over the fish and toss in a hot skillet.

282)   Codfish with mint

Preparation Time: 10 minutes   **Cooking Time**: 6 minutes   **Servings: 4**

Ingredients:
- ✓ 1 tablespoon avocado oil
- ✓ 1 tablespoon of lemon juice
- ✓ 1 tablespoon chopped mint

Directions:
- ❖ Heat a skillet with the oil over medium heat, add the mint and cod.

Ingredients:
- ✓ 1 lb cod fillet
- ✓ 2 tablespoons water

- ❖ Cook the fish for 3 minutes per side.
- ❖ Then add water and lemon juice. Cook the cod for another 2 minutes.

283)   Steamed salmon with dill

Preparation Time: 10 minutes   **Cooking Time**:   **Servings: 4**

Ingredients:
- ✓ 2 tablespoons dill, chopped
- ✓ 1 tablespoon low-fat cream cheese
- ✓ 1 teaspoon of chili flakes

Directions:
- ❖ Combine all ingredients in the bowl and mix thoroughly until smooth.

Ingredients:
- ✓ 1 pound of steamed salmon, chopped
- ✓ 1 red onion, diced

284)   Cod in tomatoes

Preparation Time: 10 minutes   **Cooking Time**: 10 minutes   **Servings: 2**

Ingredients:
- ✓ 2 tablespoons of avocado oil
- ✓ ½ teaspoon of minced garlic
- ✓ ½ cup of water

Directions:
- ❖ Heat the oil in a skillet over medium-high heat, add the garlic and fish, and cook on each side for 3 minutes.

Ingredients:
- ✓ 4 cod fillets, boneless
- ✓ 1 cup plum tomatoes, chopped
- ✓ 1 teaspoon shallot, chopped
- ❖ Then add the remaining ingredients with the fish and simmer for another ten minutes.

285)   Halibut with spinach

Preparation Time: 10 minutes   **Cooking Time**: 3 minutes   **Servings: 2**

Ingredients:
- ✓ 4 halibut fillets
- ✓ 2 tablespoons of blended spinach

Directions:
- ❖ Melt the margarine in the skillet and add the fish fillets.

Ingredients:
- ✓ 1 teaspoon margarine

- ❖ Cook them for 3 minutes per side.
- ❖ Top the cooked halibut with the spinach.

286)   Salmon and corn salad

Preparation Time: 10 minutes   **Cooking Time**: 5 minutes   **Servings: 3**

Ingredients:

✓ 2 tablespoons of canola oil
✓ ½ teaspoon of lemon juice
✓ 1 cup of corn kernels, cooked

Ingredients:

✓ 1 pound salmon, canned, shredded
✓ 1 tablespoon shallot, chopped

Directions:

❖ Place all ingredients in bowl and toss salad.

287)   Tuna salad with mustard

Preparation Time: 10 minutes   **Cooking Time**: 10 minutes   **Servings: 2**

Ingredients:

✓ ½ teaspoon of lemon juice
✓ 1 tablespoon of mustard
✓ ¼ teaspoon cayenne pepper

Directions:

❖ On medium-high pressure, pressure a skillet with oil, add salmon and roast for 5 minutes.

Ingredients:

✓ ¼ cup chickpeas, cooked
✓ 5 ounces canned albacore tuna in water, drained
✓ 1 teaspoon of olive oil
❖ Apply the capers and milk and sauté the meat over medium heat for 10 minutes. 1. In a large dish, combine the olive oil, mustard and lemon juice.
❖ In salad bowl, combine all remaining ingredients and finish with mustard mixture. Shake well with salad.

288)   Tuna with shallots

Preparation Time: 10 minutes   **Cooking Time**: 7 minutes   **Servings: 4**

Ingredients:

✓ 1 lb. tuna fillet, chopped
✓ 1 tablespoon of olive oil
✓ ½ cup shallots, chopped

Directions:

❖ Heat a skillet with oil over medium-high heat; add shallots and sauté for 3 minutes.
❖ Add the fish and cook for 4 minutes on each side.

Ingredients:

✓ 2 tablespoons of lime juice
✓ ½ cup of water

❖ Then sprinkle the fish with lime juice and water.
❖ Close the lid and simmer the tuna for 3 minutes.

289)   Cod Relish

Preparation Time: 10 minutes   **Cooking Time**: 7 minutes   **Servings: 2**

Ingredients:

✓ 1 teaspoon of dried oregano
✓ 1 cup green peas, cooked
✓ 1 onion, diced

Directions:

❖ Heat a skillet over medium-high heat with 1 tablespoon oil, add cod fillets and cook on each side for 2 minutes.
❖ After that, place the fish on serving plates.

Ingredients:

✓ 3 tablespoons of olive oil
✓ ½ teaspoon of white pepper
✓ 1 lb cod fillet, chopped
❖ Mix all remaining products and shale well in the mixing bowl.
❖ Top the onion mixture with the cod.

290) Five-spice sole

Preparation Time: 10 minutes   **Cooking Time**: 15 minutes   **Servings: 4**

Ingredients:
- ✓ 3 fillets of sole
- ✓ 1 tablespoon of five-spice seasonings

Directions:
- ❖ Rub the sole fillets with the seasonings.
- ❖ Then heat the coconut oil in the pan for 2 minutes.

Ingredients:
- ✓ 1 tablespoon of coconut oil

- ❖ Place the sole fillets in the hot oil and cook for 4.5 minutes per side.

291) Stewed clams

Preparation Time: 10 minutes   **Cooking Time**: 10 minutes   **Servings: 4**

Ingredients:
- ✓ 1 pound of clams
- ✓ 1 teaspoon of dried thyme
- ✓ 1 teaspoon ground paprika

Directions:
- ❖ Place the dried thyme, paprika and cream on the ground.
- ❖ Bring to a boil with the liquid.
- ❖ Next, apply the lemon juice and whisk well into the mixture.

Ingredients:
- ✓ ½ cup light, low-fat cream.
- ✓ 1 tablespoon of lemon juice

- ❖ Cover the lid and apply the clams.
- ❖ Simmer the stewed clams for 5 minutes.

292) Salmon with capers

Preparation Time: 10 minutes   **Cooking Time**: 15 minutes   **Servings: 4**

Ingredients:
- ✓ 2 tablespoons of avocado oil
- ✓ 1 lb salmon fillet, chopped

Directions:
- ❖ Heat a skillet with oil over medium-high heat, add the salmon and roast for 5 minutes.

Ingredients:
- ✓ 1 tablespoon capers, drained
- ✓ ½ cup low-fat milk
- ❖ Add the capers and milk and sauté the meat for 10 minutes over medium heat.

293) Horseradish cod

Preparation Time: 10 minutes   **Cooking Time**: 5 minutes   **Servings: 4**

Ingredients:
- ✓ 1 tablespoon avocado oil
- ✓ 12 ounces of cod fillet
- ✓ ½ cup of low-fat cream cheese

Directions:
- ❖ Heat a skillet with oil over medium-high heat, add cod, season with black pepper and cook for 5 minutes on each side.

Ingredients:
- ✓ ¼ teaspoon ground black pepper
- ✓ 2 tablespoons dill, chopped
- ✓ 1 tablespoon horseradish
- ❖ In a bowl, combine the cream cheese with the dill and horseradish.
- ❖ Top the cooked cod with horseradish mixture.

294) Prawns puttanesca style

Preparation Time: 10 minutes   **Cooking Time**: 10 minutes   **Servings: 4**

Ingredients:

- ✓ 5 ounces of shrimp, shelled
- ✓ 1 teaspoon of chili flakes
- ✓ ½ onion, diced
- ✓ 1 tablespoon of coconut oil

Directions:

- ❖ Heat the coconut oil in the saucepan.
- ❖ Add the shrimp and chili flakes. Cook the shrimp for 4 minutes.

Ingredients:

- ✓ 1 teaspoon garlic, diced
- ✓ 1 cup tomatoes, chopped
- ✓ ¼ cup olives, sliced
- ✓ ¼ cup of water
- ❖ Stir well and add the diced onion, garlic, tomatoes, olives and water.
- ❖ Close the lid and sauté the meat for 15 minutes.

295) Curried Snapper

Preparation Time: 10 minutes   **Cooking Time**: 10 minutes   **Servings: 4**

Ingredients:

- ✓ 1 lb snapper fillet, chopped
- ✓ 1 teaspoon of curry powder
- ✓ 1 cup celery stalk, chopped

Directions:

- ❖ Roast the snapper fillet in the olive oil for 2 minutes per side.
- ❖ Then add the celery stalk, curry powder, low-fat yogurt and water.

Ingredients:

- ✓ ½ cup low-fat yogurt
- ✓ ¼ cup of water
- ✓ 1 tablespoon of olive oil
- ❖ Stir in the fish until smooth.
- ❖ Close the lid and cook the fish over medium heat for 10 minutes.

296) Grouper with tomato sauce

Preparation Time: 10 minutes   **Cooking Time**: 10 minutes   **Servings: 4**

Ingredients:

- ✓ 12 ounces of grouper, chopped
- ✓ 2 cups grape tomatoes, chopped
- ✓ 1 hot pepper, chopped

Directions:

- ❖ Place the margarine in the saucepan.
- ❖ Add chopped grouper and sprinkle with ground cilantro.
- ❖ Roast the fish for 2 minutes per side.

Ingredients:

- ✓ 1 tablespoon margarine
- ✓ 1 teaspoon of ground coriander

- ❖ Then add the grape tomatoes and chili.
- ❖ Mix the ingredients well and close the lid.
- ❖ Cook the meal for 10 minutes over low heat.

297)   Braised sea bass

Preparation Time: 10 minutes   **Cooking Time**: 15 minutes   **Servings: 2**

Ingredients:

- ✓ 10 oz sea bass fillet
- ✓ 1 cup tomatoes, chopped
- ✓ 1 yellow onion, sliced

Directions:

- ❖ Heat skillet with olive oil.
- ❖ Add the sea bass fillet and roast on each side for 4 minutes.
- ❖ Remove the cod and add the sliced onion from the pan.
- ❖ For 2 minutes, cook.

Ingredients:

- ✓ 1 tablespoon avocado oil
- ✓ 1 teaspoon of ground black pepper

- ❖ Include the tomatoes and ground black pepper afterwards.
- ❖ Bring the mixture to a boil.
- ❖ Close the lid and add the fried sea bass.
- ❖ For 15 minutes, prepare dinner.

298)   Basil Halibut

Preparation Time: 10 minutes   **Cooking Time**: 10 minutes   **Servings: 4**

Ingredients:

- ✓ 1 pound halibut, chopped
- ✓ 1 tablespoon of dried basil

Directions:

- ❖ In a skillet, add the olive oil and heat it up.
- ❖ Meanwhile, combine the halibut, dried basil and minced garlic.

Ingredients:

- ✓ 1 teaspoon garlic powder
- ✓ 2 tablespoons of olive oil
- ❖ Add the fish to the hot oil and cook on each side for 3 minutes.

299)   Tilapia Veracruz

Preparation Time: 10 minutes   **Cooking Time**: 10 minutes   **Servings: 4**

Ingredients:

- ✓ 1 cup tomatoes, chopped
- ✓ 1 teaspoon of dried oregano
- ✓ 1 onion, diced
- ✓ ½ cup bell bell pepper, chopped

Directions:

- ❖ Heat the olive oil in the skillet and add the tilapia fillets.
- ❖ Roast the fish for 4 minutes per side. Remove the fish from the pan.
- ❖ Add the onion to the skillet and cook for 2 minutes.

Ingredients:

- ✓ ¼ cup of water
- ✓ 1 tablespoon of olive oil
- ✓ 4 tilapia fillets

- ❖ Then add the peppers, oregano and tomatoes. Mix the ingredients well and cook for 5 minutes.
- ❖ After this, add the water and fish.
- ❖ Close the lid and cook the meal for another 5 minutes.

300)   Lemon swordfish

Preparation Time: 10 minutes   **Cooking Time**: 9 minutes   **Servings: 4**

Ingredients:
- ✓ 18 ounces of swordfish fillets
- ✓ 1 tablespoon margarine
- ✓ 1 teaspoon of lemon peel
- ✓ 3 tablespoons of lemon juice

Directions:
- ❖ Cut the fish into 4 portions.
- ❖ After this, mix the lemon zest, lemon juice, ground black pepper and olive oil in the bowl. Add the minced garlic.
- ❖ Rub the fish fillets with the lemon mixture.

Ingredients:
- ✓ 1 teaspoon of ground black pepper
- ✓ 2 tablespoons of olive oil
- ✓ ½ teaspoon of minced garlic

- ❖ Grease the baking dish with margarine and arrange the swordfish fillets.
- ❖ Bake the fish for 25 minutes at 390F.

301)   Spicy scallops

Preparation Time: 10 minutes   **Cooking Time**: 10 minutes   **Servings: 4**

Ingredients:
- ✓ 1 pound of scallops
- ✓ 1 teaspoon of Cajun seasoning

Directions:
- ❖ Rub the scallops with the Cajun seasonings.
- ❖ Heat the olive oil in the skillet.

Ingredients:
- ✓ 1 tablespoon of olive oil

- ❖ Add scallops and cook for 2 minutes per side.

302)   Sole with herbs

Preparation Time: 10 minutes   **Cooking Time**: 10 minutes   **Servings: 4**

Ingredients:
- ✓ 10 oz fillet of sole
- ✓ 2 tablespoons margarine
- ✓ 1 tablespoon of dill

Directions:
- ❖ In the skillet, toss the margarine.
- ❖ Add the cumin seeds and grow with the dill.
- ❖ For 30 seconds, boil the mixture and cook it.

Ingredients:
- ✓ 1 teaspoon garlic powder
- ✓ ½ teaspoon of cumin seeds

- ❖ Then slice 2 portions of the single fillet and sprinkle with garlic powder.
- ❖ In the melted margarine mixture, place the fish fillets.
- ❖ Cook the fish on both sides for 3 minutes.

303)   Salmon with rosemary

Preparation Time: 10 minutes   **Cooking Time**: 10 minutes   **Servings: 4**

Ingredients:
- ✓ Salmon fillet 1 lb
- ✓ 4 teaspoons of olive oil

Directions:
- ❖ Cut the salmon fillet into 4 portions.
- ❖ Then rub the fillets with olive oil, lemon juice and dried rosemary.

Ingredients:
- ✓ 4 teaspoons of lemon juice
- ✓ 1 tablespoon of dried rosemary
- ❖ Place the salmon on the tray and cook for 12 minutes at 400F.

304) Zucchini boats stuffed with tuna fish

Preparation Time: 10 minutes   **Cooking Time**: 10 minutes   **Servings**: 4

Ingredients:
- ✓ 1 zucchini, blunt
- ✓ 6 ounces of tuna, canned
- ✓ 2 ounces of low-fat cheese, shredded

Directions:
- ❖ Cut zucchini in half and scoop out zucchini flesh to make zucchini boats.
- ❖ Fill zucchini boats with tuna and shredded cheese.

Ingredients:
- ✓ 1 teaspoon of chili flakes
- ✓ 1 teaspoon of olive oil

- ❖ Drizzle the zucchini with olive oil and transfer to the oven.
- ❖ Bake the meal at 385F for 20 minutes.

305) Baked cod

Preparation Time: 10 minutes   **Cooking Time**: 10 minutes   **Servings**: 4

Ingredients:
- ✓ 10 ounces of cod fillet
- ✓ 1 teaspoon of Italian seasonings

Directions:
- ❖ Rub the baking sheet with margarine.
- ❖ Then cut up the cod and sprinkle with the Italian seasonings.

Ingredients:
- ✓ 1 tablespoon margarine

- ❖ Place the fish in the baking dish and cover with aluminum foil.
- ❖ Bake the meal at 375F for 30 minutes.

306) Tuna and pineapple kebob

Preparation Time: 10 minutes   **Cooking Time**: 10 minutes   **Servings**: 4

Ingredients:
- ✓ Tuna fillet 12 oz
- ✓ 8 ounces of pineapple, peeled

Directions:
- ❖ In medium cubes, cut tuna and pineapple and brush with olive oil and ground fennel.

Ingredients:
- ✓ 1 teaspoon of olive oil
- ✓ ¼ teaspoon of ground fennel
- ❖ Then thread them through the skewers and place them on the grill at 400F in the preheated one.
- ❖ Cook the skewers on both sides for 4 minutes.

307) Paprika Tilapia

Preparation Time: 10 minutes   **Cooking Time**: 10 minutes   **Servings**: 4

Ingredients:
- ✓ 2 tilapia fillets
- ✓ 1 teaspoon ground paprika

Directions:
- ❖ Sprinkle tilapia fillets with paprika and chili powder.

Ingredients:
- ✓ ½ teaspoon of chili powder
- ✓ 2 tablespoons of avocado oil
- ❖ Then heat the avocado oil for 2 minutes in a skillet.
- ❖ Place the fish fillets in the hot oil and cook each side for 3 minutes.

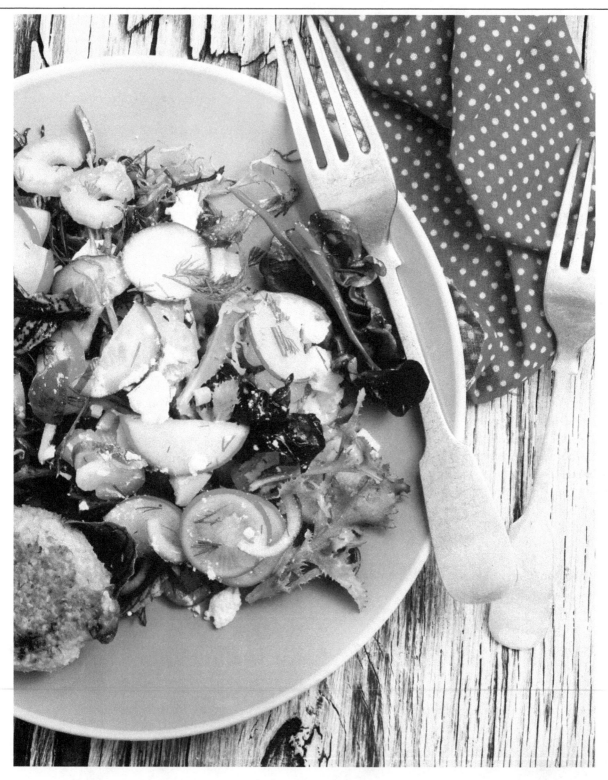

308)   Rice Soup

Preparation Time: 10 minutes   **Cooking Time**: 25 minutes   **Servings: 4**

Ingredients:
- ✓ 1 carrot, chopped
- ✓ ½ cup white rice
- ✓ 5 cups of water

Directions:
- ❖ Preheat the casserole dish well and add the olive oil.
- ❖ Then add the chicken fillet and carrot. Roast the ingredients for 5-6 minutes. Stir occasionally.

Ingredients:
- ✓ 5 ounces of chicken fillet, minced
- ✓ 1 tablespoon of olive oil
- ✓ 1 teaspoon of dried oregano
- ❖ After this, add the rice, dried oregano and water.
- ❖ Close the lid and cook the soup for 15 minutes over medium heat.

309)   Couscous soup

Preparation Time: 10 minutes   **Cooking Time**: 20 minutes   **Servings: 4**

Ingredients:
- ✓ 4 cups of water
- ✓ 1 bell pepper, chopped
- ✓ 1 onion, diced

Directions:
- ❖ Pour the olive oil into the skillet and add the diced onion. Roast the onion for 2-3 minutes per side.
- ❖ Then add the bell bell pepper and chili flakes.

Ingredients:
- ✓ 2 tablespoons of olive oil
- ✓ 1 teaspoon of chili flakes
- ✓ 1 cup of couscous
- ❖ Add the water and bring the mixture to a boil. Simmer the soup for 5 minutes.
- ❖ After this, remove it from the heat and add the couscous. Close the lid.
- ❖ Allow the soup to rest for 5 minutes.

310)   Cold cucumber soup

Preparation Time: 10 minutes   **Cooking Time**:   **Servings: 4**

Ingredients:
- ✓ 3 cucumbers, grated
- ✓ 2 cups of water

Directions:
- ❖ Mix the water with the rice milk.

Ingredients:
- ✓ 2 cups of rice milk
- ✓ 1 tablespoon of dried dill
- ❖ Then add the dried dill and grated cucumbers.
- ❖ Mix soup well and pour into bowls.

311)   Shiitake mushroom soup

Preparation Time: 10 minutes   **Cooking Time**: 25 minutes   **Servings: 6**

Ingredients:
- ✓ 8 ounces of shiitake mushrooms, chopped
- ✓ 1 onion, diced
- ✓ 1 cup cauliflower, chopped

Directions:
- ❖ Preheat the saucepan well. Add the olive oil.
- ❖ Then add the shiitake mushrooms and roast them for 2 minutes per side.

Ingredients:
- ✓ 6 cups of water
- ✓ 1 tablespoon of olive oil
- ✓ 1 teaspoon of dried oregano
- ❖ After this, add the onion and dried oregano. Roast the ingredients for 2-3 minutes.
- ❖ Then add the cauliflower and water.
- ❖ Cook the soup for an additional 15 minutes.

312)   Shallot and okra soup

Preparation Time: 10 minutes   **Cooking Time**: 25 minutes   **Servings: 4**

Ingredients:

- ✓ 10 ounces okra, chopped
- ✓ 1 carrot, diced
- ✓ 1 onion, diced

Directions:

- ❖ Place the chicken in the skillet. Add the water.
- ❖ Boil the chicken for 10 minutes.

Ingredients:

- ✓ 1 oz shallot, chopped
- ✓ 5 cups of water
- ✓ 7 ounces of chicken fillet, minced
- ❖ Then add the onion, carrot and okra. Simmer the soup for another 10 minutes.
- ❖ Add the scallions and cook the soup for another 5 minutes.

313)   Coriander Soup

Preparation Time: 10 minutes   **Cooking Time**: 20 minutes   **Servings: 4**

Ingredients:

- ✓ 8 ounces of Brussels sprouts, chopped
- ✓ 1 teaspoon of ground coriander
- ✓ 1 teaspoon of dried parsley

Directions:

- ❖ Preheat the skillet well and add the olive oil.
- ❖ Add zucchini and roast for 1 minute per side.

Ingredients:

- ✓ 5 cups of water
- ✓ 1 cup zucchini, chopped
- ✓ 1 tablespoon of olive oil
- ❖ Then add the dried parsley, ground cilantro and Brussels sprouts.
- ❖ Add the water and cook the soup over medium heat for 10 minutes.

314)   Dumpling soup with chicken

Preparation Time: 10 minutes   **Cooking Time**: 35 minutes   **Servings: 4**

Ingredients:

- ✓ 2 tablespoons of olive oil
- ✓ ½ cup white flour
- ✓ 1 teaspoon salt
- ✓ 12 ounces of chicken breast, skinless, boneless, chopped

Directions:

- ❖ In bowl mix ¼ cup water with white flour and olive oil. Knead the dough.
- ❖ Meanwhile, pour the remaining water into the saucepan and add the chicken. Simmer the ingredients for 15 minutes.

Ingredients:

- ✓ 1 teaspoon of dried dill
- ✓ 1 teaspoon of ground coriander
- ✓ 6 cups of water

- ❖ Meanwhile, make dumplings from the dough and put in the boiled chicken mixture.
- ❖ Add all remaining ingredients and close the lid.
- ❖ Simmer the soup for 10 minutes over medium heat.

315) Vegetable soup with beef

Preparation Time: 10 minutes   **Cooking Time**: 35 minutes   **Servings: 4**

Ingredients:

- ✓ 12 ounces of roast beef, minced
- ✓ 2 tablespoons of olive oil
- ✓ 1 cup broccoli, chopped

Directions:

- ❖ Mix the water with the beef and boil the ingredients for 25 minutes over medium heat.

Ingredients:

- ✓ 2 garlic cloves, diced
- ✓ 1 teaspoon of ground coriander
- ✓ 6 cups of water
- ❖ After this, add the olive oil, garlic, broccoli and cilantro. Gently stir the soup and close the lid.
- ❖ Cook the meal over medium heat for 10 minutes.

316) Noodle Soup

Preparation Time: 10 minutes   **Cooking Time**: 20 minutes   **Servings: 4**

Ingredients:

- ✓ 6 ounces of dough
- ✓ 5 cups of water
- ✓ 1 onion, diced

Directions:

- ❖ Preheat the oil in the casserole dish.
- ❖ Add the zucchini and onion. Roast the ingredients for 4-5 minutes over medium heat. Stir occasionally.

Ingredients:

- ✓ 1 zucchini, chopped
- ✓ 1 tablespoon of olive oil
- ✓ ¼ teaspoon of chilli flakes
- ❖ After this, add the chili flakes, pasta and water.
- ❖ Close the lid and cook the soup over medium heat for 10 minutes.

317) Southwest Soup

Preparation Time: 10 minutes   **Cooking Time**: 20 minutes   **Servings: 4**

Ingredients:

- ✓ 1 green chili pepper, chopped
- ✓ 1 onion, diced
- ✓ ½ clove of garlic, diced

Directions:

- ❖ Pour the olive oil into the casserole dish.
- ❖ Add the onion and garlic. Roast the vegetables for 2-3 minutes.

Ingredients:

- ✓ 8 ounces of chicken fillet, minced
- ✓ 6 cups of water
- ✓ 1 teaspoon of olive oil
- ❖ Then add the green chili and the shredded chicken.
- ❖ Add water.
- ❖ Close the lid and cook the soup over medium heat for 20 minutes.

318) Cabbage Soup

Preparation Time: 10 minutes   **Cooking Time**: 25 minutes   **Servings: 4**

Ingredients:

- ✓ 1 teaspoon ground turmeric
- ✓ 1 teaspoon of ground coriander
- ✓ 2 cups of cabbage, shredded
- ✓ 6 cups of water

Directions:

- ❖ Pour the olive oil into the casserole dish.
- ❖ Add the cauliflower and cabbage. Mix ingredients thoroughly and roast for 2-3 minutes per side.

Ingredients:

- ✓ 1 teaspoon of dried oregano
- ✓ ½ cup cauliflower, shredded
- ✓ 2 tablespoons of olive oil

- ❖ Then add all the remaining ingredients and mix thoroughly.
- ❖ Close the lid and cook the soup over medium heat for 20 minutes.

319) Broccoli soup

Preparation Time: 10 minutes   **Cooking Time**: 20 minutes   **Servings: 4**

Ingredients:

- ✓ 7 ounces of chicken fillet, minced
- ✓ 3 cups broccoli, chopped
- ✓ 6 cups of water

Directions:

- ❖ Pour the olive oil into the casserole dish and preheat it.
- ❖ Add chicken and roast for 2 minutes per side.

Ingredients:

- ✓ 1 teaspoon ground paprika
- ✓ 1 tablespoon of olive oil
- ✓ ½ bell pepper, chopped
- ❖ Then add the broccoli, ground paprika and bell bell pepper. Mix the mixture well.
- ❖ Add the water and close the lid.
- ❖ Cook the soup over medium heat for 15 minutes.

320) Carrot soup

Preparation Time: 10 minutes   **Cooking Time**: 25 minutes   **Servings: 4**

Ingredients:

- ✓ 1 cup grated carrots
- ✓ 1 onion, diced
- ✓ 3 tablespoons of olive oil

Directions:

- ❖ Pour the olive oil into the casserole dish and preheat it well.
- ❖ Add the onion and carrot. Roast the vegetables well.

Ingredients:

- ✓ 1 teaspoon of dried oregano
- ✓ 1 teaspoon of chili flakes
- ✓ 5 cups of water
- ❖ Add the chili flakes and dried oregano.
- ❖ Add the water and cook the soup over medium heat for 15 minutes.
- ❖ Then leave it for 5 minutes to rest.

321)   Rocket Soup

Preparation Time: 10 minutes   **Cooking Time**: 20 minutes   **Servings: 4**

Ingredients:
- ✓ 2 cups arugula, chopped
- ✓ 1 cup of rice milk
- ✓ 3 cups of water

Directions:
- ❖ Pour the olive oil into the casserole dish and preheat it.
- ❖ Add onion and roast until light brown.

Ingredients:
- ✓ 1 onion, diced
- ✓ 1 tablespoon of olive oil
- ✓ 1 teaspoon of chili flakes
- ❖ After this, add the arugula, chili flakes and rice milk. Mix the mixture well.
- ❖ Add the water and cook the soup for 10 minutes over medium heat.

322)   Ginger soup and Brussels sprouts

Preparation Time: 10 minutes   **Cooking Time**: 20 minutes   **Servings: 4**

Ingredients:
- ✓ 1 cup of Brussels sprouts
- ✓ 1 teaspoon ground ginger
- ✓ 1 carrot, diced

Directions:
- ❖ Pour the oil into the saucepan and preheat until hot.
- ❖ Add the carrot and roast for 1 minute per side.

Ingredients:
- ✓ 1 tablespoon of olive oil
- ✓ 1 tablespoon of dried parsley
- ✓ 5 cups of water
- ❖ After this, add the Brussels sprouts and cook the ingredients for another 2-3 minutes.
- ❖ Then add all the remaining ingredients and cook for 10 minutes over medium heat.

323)   Tarragon and shrimp soup

Preparation Time: 10 minutes   **Cooking Time**: 25 minutes   **Servings: 4**

Ingredients:
- ✓ 1 teaspoon of dried tarragon
- ✓ 1 bell pepper, chopped
- ✓ 1 tablespoon of olive oil

Directions:
- ❖ Pour the olive oil into the saucepan, add the bell bell pepper and roast it for 1 minute per side.

Ingredients:
- ✓ 5 cups of water
- ✓ 12 ounces of shrimp, shelled
- ✓ ¼ teaspoon of dried thyme
- ❖ Add the dried tarragon, shrimp and dried thyme. Stir ingredients together and cook for 4 more minutes.
- ❖ Then add the water and close the lid.
- ❖ Cook the soup over medium heat for 15 minutes.

324)   Chicken and onion soup

Preparation Time: 10 minutes   **Cooking Time**: 25 minutes   **Servings: 4**

Ingredients:

- ✓ 3 ounces spring onions, chopped
- ✓ 10 ounces of chicken fillet, minced

Directions:

- ❖ Pour the water into the saucepan, add the chicken and chili flakes. Simmer the ingredients for 15 minutes.

Ingredients:

- ✓ 6 cups of water
- ✓ 1 teaspoon of chili flakes
- ❖ Then add the spring onions and close the lid.
- ❖ Cook the soup for 10 minutes over medium heat.

325)   Basil and shrimp soup

Preparation Time: 10 minutes   **Cooking Time**: 20 minutes   **Servings: 4**

Ingredients:

- ✓ 1 teaspoon of dried basil
- ✓ 12 ounces of shrimp, shelled
- ✓ ½ carrot, chopped

Directions:

- ❖ Place all ingredients in the casserole dish.

Ingredients:

- ✓ 1 teaspoon of dried parsley
- ✓ 4 cups of water

- ❖ Close the lid and simmer the soup over medium heat for 15 minutes.

326)   Spaghetti and cabbage soup

Preparation Time: 5 minutes   **Cooking Time**: 20 minutes   **Servings: 4**

Ingredients:

- ✓ 1 cup white cabbage, chopped
- ✓ 4 ounces of dough
- ✓ 5 cups of water

Directions:

- ❖ Pour the olive oil into the saucepan and preheat it until hot.
- ❖ Then add the onion and roast until golden brown.

Ingredients:

- ✓ 1 onion, diced
- ✓ 1 tablespoon of olive oil
- ✓ ½ teaspoon of dried rosemary
- ❖ After this, add all the remaining ingredients and close the lid.
- ❖ Cook the soup over medium heat for 15 minutes.

327)   Cucumber soup

Preparation Time: 10 minutes   **Cooking Time**:   **Servings: 6**

Ingredients:

- ✓ 6 cups of rice milk
- ✓ 1 teaspoon of chili powder

Directions:

- ❖ Mix rice milk with chili powder and grated cucumber.

Ingredients:

- ✓ 3 cucumbers, grated

- ❖ Pour mixture into bowls and refrigerate for 10 minutes before serving.

328) Cream of zucchini soup

Preparation Time: 10 minutes   **Cooking Time**: 25 minutes   **Servings: 4**

Ingredients:

- ✓ 2 cups of rice milk
- ✓ 2 zucchini, grated
- ✓ 1 tablespoon of olive oil
- ✓ 1 clove of garlic, diced

Ingredients:

- ✓ ½ cup cauliflower, chopped
- ✓ 4 cups of water
- ✓ 1 teaspoon of dried thyme

Directions:

- ❖ Pour the olive oil into the saucepan, add the garlic and roast for 2-3 minutes over medium heat.
- ❖ Then add the cauliflower, dried thyme and zucchini. Add the rice milk and mix the mixture thoroughly

- ❖ Add the water and boil for 5 minutes.
- ❖ Then blend the soup with the help of the immersion blender and cook it for 5 more minutes.

329) Green bean soup with paprika

Preparation Time: 10 minutes   **Cooking Time**: 40 minutes   **Servings: 4**

Ingredients:

- ✓ 1 teaspoon ground paprika
- ✓ 10 ounces of chopped green beans
- ✓ 7 ounces of beef sirloin, minced
- ✓ 1 tablespoon of olive oil

Ingredients:

- ✓ 1 teaspoon of dried dill
- ✓ 1 cup of rice milk
- ✓ 4 cups of water

Directions:

- ❖ Pour the olive oil into the saucepan, add the beef loin and roast the meat for 5 minutes over medium heat. Stir occasionally.

- ❖ After this, add the dried dill, green beans and ground paprika.
- ❖ Add the rice milk and water.
- ❖ Close the lid and simmer the soup for 30 minutes.

330) Chicken Soup

Preparation Time: 10 minutes   **Cooking Time**: 30 minutes   **Servings: 4**

Ingredients:

- ✓ 10 ounces of chicken fillet, minced
- ✓ 2 ounces shallot, chopped

Ingredients:

- ✓ 6 cups of water
- ✓ 1 teaspoon of dried sage

Directions:

- ❖ Pour the water into the saucepan, add the dried sage and chicken.

- ❖ Cook the mixture for 20 minutes over low heat.
- ❖ Pour soup into bowls and top with scallions.

331) Onion Soup

Preparation Time: 10 minutes   **Cooking Time**: 30 minutes   **Servings: 4**

Ingredients:

- ✓ 2 onions, diced
- ✓ 1 cup of rice milk
- ✓ ½ teaspoon ground nutmeg

Ingredients:

- ✓ ¼ teaspoon ground cinnamon
- ✓ 2 cups of water
- ✓ 1 tablespoon of olive oil
- ❖ Add the water and close the lid.

Directions:

- ❖ Mix the onion with the olive oil, ground cinnamon and ground nutmeg. Place the mixture in the

- ❖ Boil the soup for 10 minutes. Then blend the soup with the help of an immersion blender.
- ❖ Pour soup into bowls.

saucepan and cook over medium heat for 5 minutes. Stir the onion occasionally.

❖ After this, add the rice milk and stir the mixture thoroughly. Cook on low heat for another 5 minutes.

332) **Spiral Soup**

Preparation Time: 10 minutes   **Cooking Time**: 20 minutes   **Servings: 4**

Ingredients:

- ✓ 2 spiral zucchini
- ✓ 1 carrot, spiralized
- ✓ 1 onion, sliced
- ✓ 5 cups of water

Directions:

❖ Pour the water and rice milk into the pan. Add the dried thyme, chili flakes and carrot.
❖ Close the lid and simmer the soup for 10 minutes

Ingredients:

- ✓ 1 teaspoon of chili flakes
- ✓ 1 teaspoon of dried thyme
- ✓ ¼ cup of rice milk

❖ After this, add all the remaining ingredients and cook the soup for another 5 minutes.
❖ Let the soup sit for 5-8 minutes and then pour into bowls.

333) **Cream of turnip soup**

Preparation Time: 10 minutes   **Cooking Time**: 20 minutes   **Servings: 4**

Ingredients:

- ✓ 2 cups turnips, peeled, chopped
- ✓ 1 teaspoon of dried oregano
- ✓ ½ teaspoon of chili flakes

Directions:

❖ Place all ingredients in the saucepan, close the lid and cook the soup for 15 minutes.

Ingredients:

- ✓ 1 cup of rice milk
- ✓ ½ cup cauliflower, chopped
- ✓ 5 cups of water
- ❖ Then blend it with the help of an immersion blender.
- ❖ Simmer the soup for another 2-3 minutes.

334) Ground Chicken Kebab

Preparation Time: 20 minutes   **Cooking Time**: 10 minutes   **Servings: 4**

Ingredients:

- ✓ 1 cup ground chicken
- ✓ 1 bell pepper, diced
- ✓ 1 onion, diced

Directions:

❖ In mixing bowl, mix ground chicken with bell bell pepper, onion, chili and olive oil.

Ingredients:

- ✓ 1 hot pepper, diced
- ✓ 1 teaspoon of olive oil

❖ Then make 4 balls with the ground chicken mixture and thread them onto metal skewers.
❖ Grill the skewers for 4 minutes per side at 400F.

335) Garlic Soup

Preparation Time: 10 minutes   **Cooking Time**: 20 minutes   **Servings: 4**

Ingredients:
- ✓ 1 pound chicken breast, skinless, boneless, chopped
- ✓ 5 cloves of garlic, diced

Directions:
- ❖ Pour the water into the pan and add the chicken breast. Close the lid and cook the mixture for 15 minutes.

Ingredients:
- ✓ 7 cups of water
- ✓ 2 cups broccoli, chopped
- ❖ Then add the garlic and broccoli. Carefully stir the soup and cook over medium-low heat for 10 minutes.

336) Zucchini soup

Preparation Time: 10 minutes   **Cooking Time**: 10 minutes   **Servings: 4**

Ingredients:
- ✓ 2 zucchini, chopped
- ✓ 5 cups of water
- ✓ ¼ cup of rice milk
- ✓ ½ teaspoon of dried tarragon

Directions:
- ❖ Pour the olive oil into the pan and preheat it well.
- ❖ Add the onion and roast it for 2 minutes. Then stir well and cook the onion for 1 minute more.
- ❖ Add the zucchini, red pepper flakes and dried tarragon.

Ingredients:
- ✓ 1 tablespoon of olive oil
- ✓ 1 onion, diced
- ✓ ½ teaspoon of chili flakes

- ❖ Mix the mixture well with the help of the spatula.
- ❖ Then add the water and rice milk.
- ❖ Close the lid and cook the soup for 5 minutes over low heat.

337) Oregano broccoli soup

Preparation Time: 10 minutes   **Cooking Time**: 15 minutes   **Servings: 4**

Ingredients:
- ✓ 3 cups broccoli, chopped
- ✓ 1 teaspoon of dried oregano
- ✓ 1 red bell pepper, chopped

Directions:
- ❖ Pour the water into the saucepan.
- ❖ Add all remaining ingredients and close the lid.

Ingredients:
- ✓ 1 teaspoon ground nutmeg
- ✓ 5 cups of water
- ✓ ¼ cup of rice milk
- ❖ Simmer the soup for 10 minutes.
- ❖ Then blend well with the help of an immersion blender.
- ❖ Simmer the soup for another 5 minutes.

338)   Chicken fillets with shallots

Preparation Time: 10 minutes   **Cooking Time**: 16 minutes   **Servings: 4**

Ingredients:

- ✓ 3 chicken fillets
- ✓ 2 ounces shallot, chopped
- ✓ ½ cup of water

Directions:

- ❖ Cut chicken fillets into strips and sprinkle with ground paprika and canola oil.
- ❖ Place the chicken in the casserole dish and roast for 3 minutes per side.

Ingredients:

- ✓ 1 teaspoon ground paprika
- ✓ 1 tablespoon of canola oil

- ❖ After this, add the scallions and water.
- ❖ Close the lid and cook the meal over medium heat for another 10 minutes.

339)   Ground chicken cutlets

Preparation Time: 15 minutes   **Cooking Time**: 10 minutes   **Servings: 4**

Ingredients:

- ✓ 2 cups ground chicken
- ✓ 1 teaspoon ground nutmeg
- ✓ ½ teaspoon of dried parsley

Directions:

- ❖ In mixing bowl, mix ground chicken with ground nutmeg, dried parsley and onion powder.
- ❖ Make cutlets with the ground chicken mixture

Ingredients:

- ✓ ½ teaspoon of onion powder
- ✓ 1 tablespoon of canola oil

- ❖ After this, pour the canola oil into the pan and preheat it well.
- ❖ Add chicken cutlets and roast for 5 minutes per side.

340)   Aromatic boiled chicken fillet

Preparation Time: 10 minutes   **Cooking Time**: 25 minutes   **Servings: 4**

Ingredients:

- ✓ ½ teaspoon of dried sage
- ✓ ½ teaspoon of dried basil
- ✓ ½ teaspoon of dried oregano

Directions:

- ❖ Pour the water into the saucepan and add the chicken fillet.

Ingredients:

- ✓ ¼ teaspoon of dry saffron
- ✓ 1 lb chicken fillet
- ✓ 1 cup of water
- ❖ Then add all the remaining ingredients and close the lid.
- ❖ Boil the chicken over medium heat for 25 minutes.

341)   Russian style chicken balls

Preparation Time: 10 minutes   **Cooking Time**: 25 minutes   **Servings: 4**

Ingredients:

- ✓ 2 cups ground chicken
- ✓ 1 chopped onion

Directions:

- ❖ In mixing bowl, mix ground chicken with onion, egg white and carrot.

Ingredients:

- ✓ 1 egg white, beaten
- ✓ ½ cup carrot, grated

- ❖ Make small balls from the ground chicken mixture and transfer them to the tray lined with baking paper.
- ❖ Bake the chicken balls for 25 minutes at 365F.

342)   Chicken skewers with basil and garlic

Preparation Time: 10 minutes   **Cooking Time**: 6 minutes   **Servings: 4**

Ingredients:
- ✓ 1 teaspoon of olive oil
- ✓ 1 teaspoon of dried basil

Directions:
- ❖ In bowl, mix olive oil with dried basil, minced garlic and chicken.

Ingredients:
- ✓ 1 teaspoon of olive oil
- ✓ 1 teaspoon of dried basil
- ❖ Thread the chicken cubes onto the skewers.
- ❖ Grill meal at 390F for 3 minutes per side or until chicken is light brown.

343)   Chicken rice

Preparation Time: 10 minutes   **Cooking Time**: 15 minutes   **Servings: 4**

Ingredients:
- ✓ 1 onion, diced
- ✓ 12 ounces of chicken fillet, diced

Directions:
- ❖ Pour the olive oil into the pan.
- ❖ Add onion and roast for 3 minutes.

Ingredients:
- ✓ 1 tablespoon of olive oil
- ✓ ¼ teaspoon of chili powder
- ❖ After this, add the chicken fillet and chili powder.
- ❖ Mix ingredients well and cook chicken rice for 10 minutes over medium heat. Stir occasionally.

344)   Lemongrass chicken

Preparation Time: 10 minutes   **Cooking Time**: 30 minutes   **Servings: 4**

Ingredients:
- ✓ 1 teaspoon of lemongrass
- ✓ 1 pound chicken breast, skinless, boneless, chopped

Directions:
- ❖ Mix chicken breast with olive oil and dried cilantro.
- ❖ Add lemongrass.

Ingredients:
- ✓ 1 tablespoon of olive oil
- ✓ ½ teaspoon of dried coriander
- ❖ After this, place the chicken in the tray and flatten it into a layer.
- ❖ Bake the meal at 360F for 30 minutes.

345)   Chicken with broccoli

Preparation Time: 10 minutes   **Cooking Time**: 35 minutes   **Servings: 4**

Ingredients:
- ✓ 2 garlic cloves, diced
- ✓ 1 cup broccoli, chopped
- ✓ 10 ounces of chicken fillet, minced

Directions:
- ❖ Mix the broccoli with the garlic, chicken and ground cumin.
- ❖ Then add the olive oil and gently mix the ingredients once more.

Ingredients:
- ✓ 1 tablespoon of olive oil
- ✓ ½ teaspoon of ground cumin
- ❖ Place ingredients in tray in one layer.
- ❖ Bake the meal at 360F for 35 minutes.

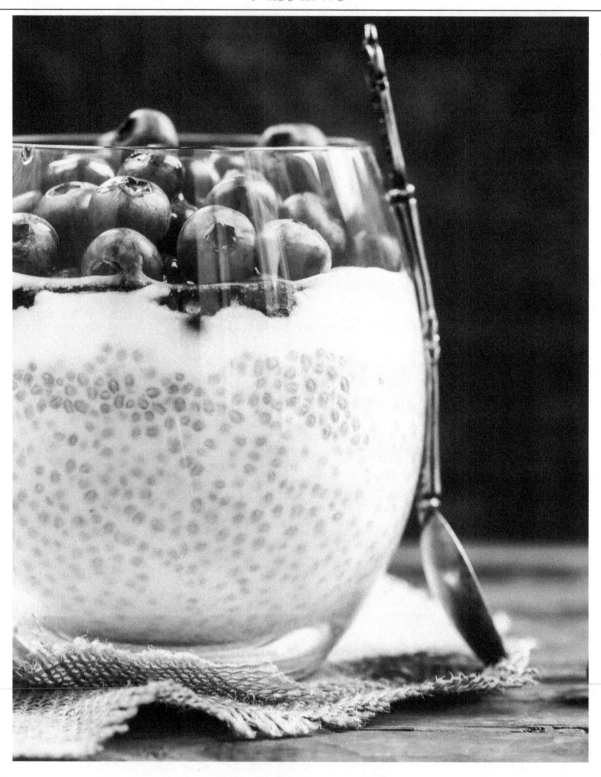

346)   Delicious peach pie

Preparation Time: 10 minutes   **Cooking Time**: 20 minutes   **Servings: 4**

Ingredients:
- ✓ Two peaches, peeled and sliced
- ✓ ½ cup of raspberries
- ✓ ½ teaspoon of coconut sugar
- ✓ Three eggs, beaten

Directions:
- ❖ In a bowl, comb the peaches with the sugar and raspberries.
- ❖ In another bowl, mix the eggs with the milk and flour and beat.

Ingredients:
- ✓ Avocado oil, 1 tablespoon
- ✓ ½ cup of almond milk
- ✓ ½ cup whole wheat flour
- ✓ ¼ cup of fat-free yogurt
- ❖ Grease a cake pan with oil, insert egg mixture, then peaches, scatter, bake at 400 degrees F for twenty minutes, slice and serve.

347)   Simple Brownies

Preparation Time: 30 minutes   **Cooking Time**: None   **Servings: 8**

Ingredients:
- ✓ Dark chocolate Six ounces, diced
- ✓ Four egg whites
- ✓ 1/2 cup of hot water
- ✓ Extract 1 teaspoon of vanilla
- ✓ 2/3 cup sugar for the coconut

Directions:
- ❖ Integrate the chocolate and hot water into a cup and shake very well.
- ❖ Apply the vanilla extract and egg whites and mix well again.
- ❖ Integrate the sugar with the flour, baking powder and nuts in another pan. Stir.

Ingredients:
- ✓ One and 1/2 full cup of flour
- ✓ 1/2 cup sliced walnuts
- ✓ Kitchen spray
- ✓ 1 tablespoon baking powder

- ❖ Combine the two mixtures, mix well, place in a cake pan greased with cooking spray, spread well, bake for 30 minutes in the oven, cool, cut and serve.

348)   Apple Tart

Preparation Time: 15 minutes   **Cooking Time**: 25 minutes   **Servings: 8**

Ingredients:
- ✓ Four apples, diced and cut into pieces
- ✓ 1/4 cup of natural apple juice
- ✓ Cranberries per 1/2 cup, dried
- ✓ Two tablespoons of cornstarch
- ✓ Two teaspoons of coconut sugar
- ✓ Extract 1 teaspoon of vanilla

Directions:
- ❖ Supplement blueberries with apple juice in a cup.
- ❖ Supplement apples with cornstarch in another pan, swirl and apply blueberry mixture.
- ❖ Mix everything together, add the vanilla and cinnamon, and then mix again.

Ingredients:
- ✓ 1/4 teaspoon dry cinnamon
  As for the crust:
- ✓ A cup and a quarter of whole wheat flour
- ✓ Two teaspoons of sugar
- ✓ Coconut oil for three teaspoons, melted
- ✓ 1/4 cup of ice water
- ❖ Sift the flour with the sugar, oil and cooled water into another bowl and mix until the dough is finished.
- ❖ Shift dough, flatten well, roll into a circle and move to a pastry pan on a workpiece surface.
- ❖ Push crust well into baking dish, pour apple mixture over crust, place in oven, bake for 25 minutes at 375 °F, and lower temperature, slice and serve.

349)   Special Victoria Sponge Cake

Preparation Time: 15-20 minutes   **Cooking Time**: 25 minutes   **Servings: 10**

Ingredients:

- ✓   50ml heavy cream
- ✓   A splash of milk (if necessary)
- ✓   250g (9oz) of self-raising flour
- ✓   4 medium eggs

Directions:

- ❖   Grease two shallow 8-inch cake pans and then line them with baking parchment. Preheat the oven to 180 degrees C (160 degrees Fan)/350 degrees F/Gas 4.
- ❖   In a large bowl, include the melted butter and sugar and whisk until very pale and fluffy. This is likely to take about 5-10 minutes. This can be achieved in a standalone mixer, if needed.
- ❖   Apply one egg and a huge spoonful of flour to the mixture and beat again. Until all the eggs are included, repeat this process. Sift out the excess flour and then use a wide metal spoon to fold over the mixture.

Ingredients:

- ✓   250g (9oz) caster sugar
- ✓   250g (9oz) unsalted butter, well softened
- ✓   About 5 tablespoons of raspberry jam (add more or less for your favorite flavor)
- ❖   Add a splash of milk if the dough doesn't have a droopy consistency (i.e., it slides off a spoon quickly).
- ❖   Spread the mixture between the two pans, smooth the surface and bake for 25 minutes.
- ❖   They should stay together until the cakes have been boiled and cooled. Before soft peaks form, whip the heavy cream. Spread the jelly on one of the cakes and then spread the whipped cream on top of the jam. Place on top of the second cake and sift in the powdered sugar for decoration.

350)   Rhubarb Crumble

Preparation Time: 15 minutes   **Cooking Time**: 30 minutes   **Servings: 6**

Ingredients:

- ✓   2 tablespoons water
- ✓   2 tablespoons granulated sugar
- ✓   2 apples, peeled, cored and thinly sliced
- ✓   1 cup chopped rhubarb
- ✓   ½ cup unsalted butter, room temperature

Directions:

- ❖   Preheat the oven to about 325°F.
- ❖   Lightly oil a buttered 8-by-8-inch baking dish; set aside.
- ❖   Mix the rice, sugar and cinnamon in a small bowl until well blended.
- ❖   Rub the dough between your fingertips and apply the butter so that it resembles coarse crumbs.

Ingredients:

- ✓   ½ teaspoon ground cinnamon
- ✓   ½ cup of brown sugar
- ✓   1 cup all-purpose flour
- ✓   Unsalted butter to grease the pan.

- ❖   Mix rhubarb, apple, sugar and water in a medium saucepan over medium heat and simmer for about 20 minutes or until rhubarb is tender.
- ❖   Across the baking bowl, pour in the fruit mixture and finish with the crumble evenly.
- ❖   Bake for 20-30 minutes or until crumble is golden brown. Serve hot.

351) Fresh parfait

Preparation Time: 10 minutes   **Cooking Time**: None   **Servings: 6**

Ingredients:

- ✓ Four cups of fat-free yogurt
- ✓ Stevia, 3 tablespoons.
- ✓ Two tablespoons of lime juice

Directions:

- ❖ Mix the yogurt with the stevia, lime juice, lime zest and mint in a bowl and stir.

Ingredients:

- ✓ Two teaspoons of lime zest, grind
- ✓ Four grapefruits, chopped and peeled
- ✓ Cut 1 tablespoon of spices
- ❖ Divide grapefruits into small cups, add each to yogurt mixture and serve.

352) Blueberry Peach Crunch

Preparation Time: 15 minutes   **Cooking Time**: 45 minutes   **Servings: 10**

Ingredients:

- ✓ ½ cup unsalted butter
- ✓ ¾ cup packed brown sugar
- ✓ ¾ cup white flour
- ✓ 1 tablespoon freshly squeezed lemon juice

Directions:

- ❖ Preheat the oven to approximately 375°F.
- ❖ Stone the peaches and thinly divide them into 3⁄4-inch strips.
- ❖ "Spray oil on a baking sheet 12" by 9".
- ❖ Arrange the peach slices and blueberries evenly around the base of the dish

Ingredients:

- ✓ ¼ cup of sugar
- ✓ 1 cup fresh blueberries
- ✓ 7 medium peaches

- ❖ Sprinkle the fruit with lemon juice and honey.
- ❖ In a bowl, mix brown sugar and flour and butter until crumbly.
- ❖ Sprinkle the crumble combination evenly over the berries.
- ❖ Bake for about 45 minutes until the fruit has softened and the crumble is golden brown.
- ❖ Serve hot.

353) Apple Crumble

Preparation Time: 15-20 minutes   **Cooking Time**: 40-45 minutes   **Servings: 4**

Ingredients:

For your crumble
- ✓ Butter nut for greasing
- ✓ 200g (7oz) unsalted butter, diced at room temperature
- ✓ 175g (6oz) sugar
- ✓ 300g plain flour, a pinch of sifted salt

Directions:

- ❖ Preheat the oven to about 180 degrees C (160 degrees Fan)/350 degrees F/Gas 4.
- ❖ In a large bowl, place the flour and sugar and combine well. Rub many pieces of butter over the flour mixture at a time. Until the mixture resembles breadcrumbs, continue rubbing.

Ingredients:

For your stuffing
- ✓ 1 pinch of ground cinnamon
- ✓ 1 tablespoon plain flour
- ✓ 50g (2oz) sugar
- ✓ Peeled 450g (1lb) apples, coreless and cut into 1cm/½in pieces
- ❖ In a large bowl, place the fruit and sprinkle in the flour, sugar and cinnamon. Mix well and be careful not to tear the fruit.
- ❖ Butter a 24cm/9-inch baking dish. Spread the fruit mixture on the bottom, then scatter the crumble mix over the top.
- ❖ For 45-50 minutes, bake until crumble is golden brown and fruit mixture is bubbly.

354) Pavlov with peaches

Preparation Time: 30 min plus 1 hour cooling time

Cooking Time: None

Servings: 8

Ingredients:

- ✓ 2 cups canned peaches drained in juice
- ✓ ½ teaspoon of pure vanilla extract
- ✓ 1 cup superfine sugar

Directions:

- ❖ Preheat the oven to about 225°F.
- ❖ Cover parchment paper with a baking sheet; set aside.
- ❖ Beat egg whites in a large bowl for about 1 minute or until soft peaks develop.
- ❖ Beat in the cream of tartar.
- ❖ Add the sugar until the egg whites are very firm and glossy, 1 tablespoon at a time. Do not over beat the eggs.
- ❖ Now whisk in the vanilla.
- ❖ Spread the meringue evenly on the baking sheet, so that you have 8 circles.

Ingredients:

- ✓ ½ teaspoon of cream of tartar
- ✓ 4 large egg whites, at room temperature

- ❖ In the center of each circle, use the back of the spoon to make an indentation.
- ❖ For about 1 hour, bake the meringues or until a light brown crust forms.
- ❖ Turn off the oven and let the meringues rest overnight, still in the oven.
- ❖ Remove and place meringues from sheet on serving plates.
- ❖ Evenly distribute the peaches in the center of the meringues and serve.
- ❖ Place some leftover meringue in a lined jar for up to 1 week at room temperature.

355) Cooled lemon cake

Preparation Time: 5-10 minutes

Cooking Time: 45 minutes

Servings: 4

Ingredients:

- ✓ 2 cups sugar, powdered variety
- ✓ ¼ cup of lemon juice
- ✓ 1 cup of water

Directions:

- ❖ Preheat the oven to approximately 350° F.
- ❖ Grease a 13' by 9' by 2' baking dish and sift in flour.
- ❖ In a bowl, place the cake mix and combine the applesauce, beaten eggs, and water. You should blend for 30 seconds on low and then switch to medium and blend for another 2 minutes with your food processor.
- ❖ Place flour in the pan and bake until cooked (when inserted, a toothpick comes out clean), about 40 minutes.

Ingredients:

- ✓ 3 eggs
- ✓ ½ cup applesauce, unsweetened
- ✓ 1 box (18 ½ oz.) of a yellow cake mix
- ❖ Cool the cake, then leave it in the pan
- ❖ Combine the lemon juice and powdered sugar until completely mixed.
- ❖ Make slits, each 1/2 inch apart, in the top of the cake.
- ❖ Spoon the lemon glaze over the end, letting it drip into the holes
- ❖ The entire top of the cake would finally be sealed.
- ❖ Relax and work long hours and enjoy

356)   Lemon cheesecake

Preparation Time: 15 minutes   **Cooking Time**:   **Servings: 4**

Ingredients:

For the base
- ✓ 100g (3½oz) soft unsalted butter
- ✓ 200g (7oz) digestive cookies

Directions:

- ❖ Process the cookies in the mixer until they are fine crumbs, then add the butter through the spout in small pieces while the processor is still working. You can end up with a similar quality to wet dough.
- ❖ Butter a jar and firmly push the base mixture into the rim of the jar and place in the refrigerator to set.
- ❖ Beat the cream until it is thickened enough to almost hold its shape, but not quite yet. To save time, use an electronic whisk if you have one.

Ingredients:

For the dressing
- ✓ 1 single dish of cream (or whipping cream, a small dish)
- ✓ 1 packet of cream cheese (a standard packet usually around 200-300 g)
- ✓ Juice of 1 lemon
- ✓ 250g of icing sugar (sifted)
- ❖ In the cream cheese packet, beat until the mixture is smooth.
- ❖ Apply lemon juice and sifted powdered sugar and beat again until strong and thick.
- ❖ Place the topping on the base and spread it out. Return the pan to the refrigerator before the topping has formed. As preferred, include berries.

357)   Baked peaches with cream cheese

Preparation Time: 10 minutes   **Cooking Time**: 15 minutes   **Servings: 4**

Ingredients:

- ✓ 1 cup plain cream cheese, room temperature
- ✓ ½ cup crushed meringue cookies (here)
- ✓ ¼ teaspoon ground cinnamon

Directions:

- ❖ Preheat the oven to about 350°F.
- ❖ Cover parchment paper with a baking sheet; set aside.
- ❖ Mix the meringue cookies, cream cheese, cinnamon and nutmeg in a shallow dish.

Ingredients:

- ✓ Pinch of ground nutmeg
- ✓ 8 canned peach halves in juice
- ✓ 2 spoons of honey
- ❖ Spoon the cream cheese mixture generously over the halves of the cavity peaches.
- ❖ Place peaches on baking sheet and bake until fruit is soft and cheese is melted, or about 15 minutes.
- ❖ Transfer peaches to plates, 2 per individual, from baking dish and drizzle with honey before eating.

358)   Raspberry Brule

Preparation Time: 15-20 minutes   **Cooking Time**: 1 minutes   **Servings: 4**

Ingredients:

- ✓ 1 cup fresh raspberries
- ✓ ¼ teaspoon ground cinnamon
- ✓ ¼ cup of brown sugar, divided

Directions:

- ❖ Preheat the baking oven.
- ❖ Beat the heavy cream, cream cheese, 2 teaspoons brown sugar and cinnamon together in a small bowl for about 4 minutes or until very smooth and fluffy.
- ❖ Divide raspberries evenly among four ramekins (4 ounces).

Ingredients:

- ✓ ½ cup plain cream cheese, room temperature
- ✓ ½ cup light sour cream

- ❖ Spoon the cream cheese combination over the berries and smooth the tops.
- ❖ Store ramekins until ready to eat dessert in the refrigerator, sealed.
- ❖ On each ramekin, sprinkle 1/2 tablespoon brown sugar evenly.
- ❖ Place the ramekins on a baking sheet until the sugar is caramelized and golden brown, and bake them 4 inches from the heating element.
- ❖ Remove from microwave. Let them rest for 1 minute and serve rules

359)   Cherry shortbread

Preparation Time: 20 minutes   **Cooking Time**: 40 minutes   **Servings: 4**

Ingredients:

- ✓ 180g (6oz) plain flour
- ✓ 55g (2oz) of caster sugar, plus extra to finish off

Directions:

- ❖ Heat your oven to about 190°C (170°C fan)/375°F/gas 5.
- ❖ Together, beat the butter and sugar until creamy.
- ❖ To make a smooth dough, whisk in the flour.
- ❖ Apply (if using) cherries and gently stir to blend.

Ingredients:

- ✓ 125g (4oz) unsalted butter
- ✓ Optional: 2 tablespoons of glace cherries - chopped

- ❖ Turn on a work surface and gently roll out until the dough is 1 cm/1⁄2 inch deep.
- ❖ Break it into fingers or rolls and place on a baking sheet. Sprinkle with granulated sugar and chill for 20 minutes in the freezer.
- ❖ Bake for 15-20 minutes in the oven or until golden brown and pale. Set aside on a wire rack to cool.

360) Sweet cinnamon custard

Preparation Time: 20 minutes   **Cooking Time**: 1 hour   **Servings: 6**

Ingredients:

- ✓ ½ teaspoon ground cinnamon
- ✓ 1 teaspoon of pure vanilla extract
- ✓ ¼ cup granulated sugar
- ✓ 4 eggs

Directions:

- ❖ Preheat the oven to about 325°F.
- ❖ Gently grease six ramekins (4 ounces) and place in baking dish; set aside.
- ❖ Whisk together the eggs, rice milk, vanilla, sugar and cinnamon in a large bowl until you have a very creamy paste.
- ❖ In a pitcher, pour the liquid through a fine sieve.
- ❖ Evenly distribute the custard mixture among the ramekins.

Ingredients:

- ✓ 1½ cups plain rice milk
- ✓ Unsalted butter to grease the ramekins.
- ✓ Cinnamon sticks, for garnish (optional)

- ❖ Rinse the pan with hot water until the water comes halfway up the sides of the ramekins. Be careful not to get water into the ramekins.
- ❖ Bake until the creams are set and a knife inserted into the middle of one of the creams comes out clean, or about 1 hour.
- ❖ Remove the baked creams from the oven and remove the ramekins from the bath.
- ❖ Chill for 1 hour on wire racks and then move the creams to the refrigerator to chill for another hour.
- ❖ Garnish each cream, if necessary, with a cinnamon stick.

361) Honey bread pudding

Preparation Time: 15-20 minutes   **Cooking Time**: 40-45 minutes   **Servings: 4**

Ingredients:

- ✓ 6 cups of white bread cubes
- ✓ 1 teaspoon of pure vanilla extract
- ✓ ¼ cup of honey

Directions:

- ❖ Lightly oil a buttered 8-by-8-inch baking dish; set aside.
- ❖ Whisk together the rice milk, eggs, egg whites, sugar and vanilla in a medium bowl.
- ❖ Add the bread cubes and stir until covered with the bread.

Ingredients:

- ✓ 2 large egg whites
- ✓ 2 eggs
- ✓ 1½ cups plain rice milk
- ❖ Move the mixture and cover with plastic wrap in the baking dish.
- ❖ Keep the dish in the refrigerator for a minimum of 3 hours.
- ❖ Preheat the oven to 325°F.
- ❖ Remove the plastic wrap from the pan and bake the pudding for 35-40 minutes, or until a knife inserted in the middle comes out clean and golden brown.
- ❖ Serve hot.

362) Vanilla Couscous Pudding

Preparation Time: 15-20 minutes   **Cooking Time**: 20 minutes   **Servings: 4**

Ingredients:
- ✓ 1 cup of couscous
- ✓ ¼ teaspoon ground cinnamon
- ✓ ½ cup of honey

Directions:
- ❖ In a large saucepan, combine the water, rice milk and vanilla seeds over medium-low heat.
- ❖ Bring the milk to a gentle boil, reduce the heat to low and let the milk simmer for about 10 minutes to allow the vanilla flavor to enter the milk.
- ❖ Remove the saucepan from the heat.

Ingredients:
- ✓ 1 vanilla pod, separated
- ✓ ½ cup of water
- ✓ 1½ cups plain rice milk
- ❖ Pull out the vanilla pod and remove the seeds from the pod into the hot milk with the tip of a sharp knife.
- ❖ Stir in the cinnamon and sugar.
- ❖ Cover the dish, stir the couscous and let it sit for about 10 minutes.
- ❖ Using a fork, fluff the couscous before eating.

363) Victoria Sponge Cake

Preparation Time: 10 minutes   **Cooking Time**: 35 minutes   **Servings: 4**

Ingredients:
- ✓ 50ml heavy cream
- ✓ A splash of milk (if necessary)
- ✓ 250g (9oz) of self-raising flour
- ✓ 4 medium eggs

Directions:
- ❖ Grease two shallow 8-inch cake pans and then line them with baking paper for baking. Preheat the oven to 180°C (160° F) / 350°s F / Gas 4.
- ❖ In a large bowl, include the melted butter and sugar and whisk until very pale and fluffy. This is likely to take about 5-10 minutes. This can be achieved in a standalone mixer, if needed.
- ❖ Apply one egg and one giant spoonful of flour to the mixture and beat again. Until all the eggs are included, repeat this process. Sift out excess flour and then use a large metal spoon to fold over the mixture.

Ingredients:
- ✓ 250g (9oz) caster sugar
- ✓ 250g (9oz) unsalted butter, well softened
- ✓ About 5 tablespoons of raspberry jam (add more or less for your favorite flavor)
- ❖ Add a splash of milk if the dough doesn't have a droopy consistency (i.e., it slides off a spoon quickly).
- ❖ Spread the mixture between the two pans, smooth the surface and bake for 25 minutes.
- ❖ They should sandwich together until the cakes have been boiled and cooled. Whip the heavy cream until soft peaks form. Spread the jelly on one of the cakes and then spread the whipped cream on top of the jam. Place on top of the second cake and sift in the powdered sugar for decoration.

364) Desserts and snacks

Preparation Time: 5 minutes

Ingredients:
- ✓ 1/4 teaspoon of cinnamon
- ✓ 1/2 cup of almond milk
- ✓ 1 large egg

Directions:
- ❖ Twist and coarsely cut apple halves.
- ❖ In a large bowl, mix the egg, oatmeal and almond milk. Using a fork, mix well. Add the apple and cinnamon. When well combined, mix again.

Cooking Time: 5 minutes   **Servings: 1**

Ingredients:
- ✓ 1/3 cup quick-cooking oatmeal
- ✓ 1/2 medium apple

- ❖ Cook in microwave for 2 minutes, on high heat. With a fork, fluff up. If necessary, cook for an additional 30-60 seconds.
- ❖ If thinner cereal is needed, add a little more milk or water

365) Lemon and lime sorbet

Preparation Time: 5 min plus 3 hours cooling time

Ingredients:
- ✓ ½ cup heavy cream (whipping cream)
- ✓ Juice of 1 lime
- ✓ Zest of 1 lime
- ✓ ½ cup of freshly squeezed lemon juice

Directions:
- ❖ Over medium-high heat, place a large saucepan and add the water, sugar and two tablespoons of lemon zest.
- ❖ Bring the mixture to a boil and then reduce the heat for 15 minutes and simmer.

Cooking Time: 15 minutes   **Servings: 8**

Ingredients:
- ✓ 3 tablespoons of lemon zest, divided
- ✓ 1 cup granulated sugar
- ✓ 2 cups of water

- ❖ Place the mixture in a large bowl and apply a tablespoon of lemon zest, lemon juice, lime zest and lime juice to the remaining mixture.
- ❖ Chill the mixture in the refrigerator for about 3 hours before it is absolutely cold.
- ❖ Blend and strain the mixture into an ice cream maker with the heavy cream.
- ❖ Freeze according to supplier's directions.

366) Cherry Pie

Preparation Time: 10-20 minutes

Ingredients:
- ✓ 20 ounces of pie filling - cherry
- ✓ 1 teaspoon of baking soda
- ✓ 1 teaspoon baking powder
- ✓ 1 teaspoon of vanilla
- ✓ 2 cups of white flour

Directions:
- ❖ Preheat the oven to about 350°F and, at room temperature, soften the butter
- ❖ Cream the eggs, sugar, vanilla and sour cream together,
- ❖ Combine baking powder, flour, and baking soda in another dish.

Cooking Time: 45 minutes   **Servings: 24**

Ingredients:
- ✓ 1 cup of sour cream
- ✓ 1 cup of sugar
- ✓ 2 eggs
- ✓ ½ cup unsalted butter

- ❖ Gradually mix the dry ingredients into the wet cream mixture, folding to mix completely. Grease a 9' x 13' baking dish and place the batter in it.
- ❖ Layer the cherry mixture equally over the batter.
- ❖ Bake for about 40 minutes, until golden brown.

367)   Sponge pudding with syrup

Preparation Time: 15-20 minutes   **Cooking Time**: 35-40 minutes   **Servings: 4**

Ingredients:

- ✓ 6 spoons of golden syrup
- ✓ 100g (3½oz) self-raising flour
- ✓ 2 eggs

Directions:

- ❖ In a saucepan or food processor, cream the butter and sugar.
- ❖ To prevent curdling, apply one egg and gently combine with one tablespoon of flour. Add the other egg and combine thoroughly.
- ❖ Fold the flour.

Ingredients:

- ✓ 100g (3½oz) caster sugar
- ✓ 100g (3½oz) softened unsalted butter

- ❖ Measure sugar into a buttered pudding bowl. On top of sugar, spoon cake mixture.
- ❖ With a fold, cover with a buttered sheet to allow for expansion.
- ❖ Bake for 35-40 minutes at 200°C (180°C fan)/400°F/Gas 6 until a skewer comes out clean.

368)   Crunchy apple granita

Preparation Time: 15 minutes plus 4 hours freezing time   **Cooking Time**:   **Servings: 4**

Ingredients:

- ✓ ¼ cup freshly squeezed lemon juice
- ✓ 2 cups unsweetened apple juice

Directions:

- ❖ Heat the sugar and water in a medium-sized saucepan over medium-high heat.
- ❖ Bring the mixture to a boil and then reduce the heat to low and simmer for about 15 more minutes or until the liquid has reduced by half.
- ❖ Remove the pan from the heat and pour the liquid into a large, shallow metal pan.

Ingredients:

- ✓ ½ cup of water
- ✓ ½ cup granulated sugar

- ❖ For about 30 minutes, let the mixture set and then stir in the apple juice and lemon juice.
- ❖ In a freezer, place your pan.
- ❖ Run a fork through the liquid after 1 hour to break up any ice crystals that have developed. Scrape down the sides as well.
- ❖ Return the pan to the freezer and continue to stir and scrape, making the slush every 20 minutes.
- ❖ Serve once; mixture is completely frozen and appears as crushed ice after about 3 hours.

AUTHOR BIBLIOGRAPHY

THE RENAL DIET FOR HER: *120+ Kidney Friendly Recipes to Control Your Renal Disease and Avoid Dialysis. Enjoy Delicious Foods and Stay Healthy by Learning What to Eat. Manage your CKD!*

THE RENAL DIET FOR HIM: COOKBOOK FOR BEGINNERS' MEN: 120+ Low Sodium, Low Potassium Tasty Recipes to Manage Chronic Kidney Disease Properly, and Avoid Dialysis Even for Newly Diagnosed

CKD COOKBOOK: *120+ Easy, Flavorful Recipes for every stage of kidney disease! Reboot your health with these new renal-diet recipes and avoid dialysis!*

THE RENAL DIET FOR BEGINNERS: *120+ Recipes to Take Care of Your Kidneys, Without Giving Up on Taste. Prevent Kidney Failure by Eating Healthy!*

THE RENAL DIET FOR KIDS: *The Complete Guide that will help kids to Avoid Kidney Disease and Prevent Dialysis! 120+ Recipes for CKD and Renal Failure!*

THE RENAL DIET FOR COUPLE: 2 BOOKS in 1: *The Ultimate Guide to Heal Kidney Disease and Avoid Dialysis With 200+ Wholesome, Easy to Follow and Delicious Recipes!*

THE RENAL DIET FOR ATHLETE: 2 Books in 1: *The Guide for Beginners to Lose Weight Quickly and Regain Confidence! Manage Kidney Disease and Avoid Dialysis with Over 240 Healthy, Low Sodium, Low Potassium & Low Phosphorus Recipes!*

THE RENAL DIET FOR ONE: 2 Books in 1: *Cookbook for Beginners: How to Manage CKD to Escape Dialysis. RECIPES for a Progressive Renal Function Recovery! 240+ Kidney-Friendly Recipes!*

THE RENAL DIET FOR WOMEN OVER 50: 2 Books in 1: *The Ultimate and Complete Guide to Lose Weight Quickly and Regain Confidence, Cut Cholesterol and Balance Hormones at The Same Time!*

THE RENAL DIET ON A BUDGET: 2 Books in 1: *Discover how to avoid the progression of incurable kidney disease, with more than 200 flavorful Recipes Cookbook!*

THE RENAL HEALTHY DIET: 3 Books in 1: *Cookbook for beginners for newly diagnoses with kidney disease A comprehensive guide with 300+ easy and quick healthy recipes to manage Chronic Kidney Disease!*

THE RENAL DIET FOR SPORT: 3 Books in 1: *Cookbook for Beginners: Learn 350 Healthy Recipes with Low Sodium, Potassium, and Phosphorus. Don't renounce the sport! For all levels of athlete!*

CONCLUSIONS

A diet deficient in phosphorus, protein, and sodium is a renal diet. An individual's body is different, so each patient needs to work with a renal dietitian to create a diet customized to the patient's needs. A renal diet often emphasizes the value of eating high-quality protein and limiting fluids.

Therefore, individuals with kidney disease must follow a kidney-friendly diet to enjoy a healthy life.

Managing chronic kidney disease (CKD) requires lifestyle adjustments, but it may help to know you're not alone. U.S. counts mjore than 35 million people have been diagnosed with malfunctioning kidneys or are battling kidney disease. As a registered dietitian (RD) with extensive experience in helping patients take control of their kidney disease, I have helped patients manage the physical symptoms associated with this disease and deal with the emotional toll this life change can bring. Without knowing what the future holds, uncertainty, fear, depression, and anxiety can be common. It may even seem like dialysis is inevitable, and you may wonder if it is worth the time and effort to try to manage this stage of the disease or if it is even possible to delay the progression. As an expert in this field, I can assure you that it is not only possible, but yours to achieve: only 1 in 50 diagnosed with CKD ends up on dialysis. So, together and with the right tools, we can work to delay and ultimately prevent end-stage renal disease and dialysis. Success is gained through diet and lifestyle modifications. Using simple, manageable strategies, I have seen firsthand how my patients have grown stronger with the knowledge. They went on to lead whole, productive, and happy lives, continuing to work, play and spend time with their loved ones - just as it should be!

Diet is a vital part of CKD treatment and can help immensely slow the disease's progression. Some ingredients help the kidneys function, while others make them work harder. This book has focused on crowding out the unhealthy ones with the healthy and helpful ones. Also, targeting factors such as salt and carbohydrate intake is essential to reduce the risk of hypertension, diabetes, and other diseases resulting from kidney failure. I cannot stress enough the importance of consulting a dietitian during the progression of CKD to optimize health. This book is a good start, as it is designed specifically for the treatment of this population.

Adopting a kidney-friendly lifestyle can be challenging at first, but following these recipes will reduce the anxiety associated with choosing intelligent food options for your daily life. And so you don't have to worry about your new diet being restrictive or unsustainable, I want to assure you that these recipes are easy and delicious and will give you a realistic and satisfying way to make this lifestyle change. This book will guide you every step of the way. Doing so will help you take the stress of meal planning out of the equation and help you focus on the essential things in life.